BTLS ACCESS

James B. Gargan

Emergency Training Associates
Union Bridge, MD

First Edition

ISBN 1-887321-00-4

Publication design by Lou Jordan and Jack Sanders
Cover design by Lou Jordan

DEDICATION

"BTLS ACCESS" is dedicated to my partner and brother of thirty-two years, Harvey D. Grant. Harvey left us for the big firehouse in the sky on January 24, 1993.

Harvey will always be remembered as the father of EMS and vehicle rescue. For years his dream was to have ambulance crews trained in quick access to accident victims, thus enhancing the usable time of the "golden hour."

Many hours turning into years have been spent perfecting techniques and the proper tools to enable the EMT to do the job.

I hope this book will do justice to that end.

TABLE OF CONTENTS

FOREWORD

Trauma remains a major killer in our society and motor vehicle collisions continue to take the lives of thousands each year. Thousands more suffer major injuries that leave them disabled. In addition to this horrible toll, the financial cost of motor vehicle trauma runs into the millions of dollars. As a society, we have made some strides in reducing the cost in lives, with the use of seat belts and passive restraints. Design of vehicles has improved, providing increased protection after a collision. However, those same changes that protect victims and keep them inside the vehicle also make it harder for EMS and Rescue personnel to get to the victim after the accident.

Progress has also been made in improvement of care of the trauma victim. Training of prehospital personnel in Basic Trauma Life Support and the development of Trauma Systems and the education of physicians and nurses has done much to save lives and return trauma victims back to useful productive lives.

Trauma is a disease of time. The sooner that a trauma victim receives definitive surgical management of their injury, the better the change of survival. The concept of the **GOLDEN HOUR** was first put forth by Dr. R Adams Cowley and is the standard by which all of us in the prehospital environment operate. That hour begins when the victim is injured, not when we remove them from the vehicle.

Unfortunately, all too often, an EMS crew or First Responder unit arrives on the scene of a motor vehicle collision only to find themselves unable to reach the victim inside the vehicle. Precious minutes of that Golden Hour are lost, awaiting the arrival of rescue tools and personnel.

It was that "wait" and the inability of personnel to apply the training from BTLS that led Harvey Grant to develop the concept for this course. Harvey's untimely death prevented his completing this task. His long time colleague and friend, Jim Gargan picked up the "gauntlet" and came up with the "BTLS ACCESS" program.

The purpose of this course is to provide EMS crews with the training to utilize tools commonly carried on an ambulance or first responder unit to reach entrapped victims and begin stabilization and extrication, while awaiting the arrival of rescue units. This allows us to "give back" some of the Golden Hour to the person who needs it most, the patient.

To Harvey, for his many contributions to emergency care and his support of BTLS, we offer our deepest thanks. He will be sorely missed. To Jim, for his efforts in this course, our deep appreciation. To all of you who answer the call for help, thank you for caring. You do make a difference.

John E. Campbell, MD, FACEP
President

Roy L. Alson, Phd, MD, FACEP
Member Board of Directors

The First prehospital trauma course ever developed, Basic Trauma Life Support, was introduced in August of 1982. After twelve years of dedicated work by volunteer instructors from every level of emergency medicine, BTLS has become internationally accepted as the training course for prehospital trauma care. More than this, BTLS has become an international organization and network of instructors of prehospital trauma care. Basic Trauma Life Support is endorsed by the American College of Emergency Physicians and the National Association of EMS Physicians. Each local chapter is represented at the annual international meetings. The purpose of the organization is to foster trauma training and maintain up-to-date high standards for the BTLS Advanced, Pediatric BTLS and BTLS Access courses, for further information phone 1-800-495-2857.

PREFACE

Many books have already been written on the subject of "vehicle rescue" and many more will be, however, this is **not** one of them. Vehicle rescue, when addressed properly, shows many options for accomplishing all tasks concerning the subject. "BTLS ACCESS" is aimed at the two man medic team who must quickly and safely gain access into a wrecked vehicle, treat, disentangle, package and hopefully, remove and transport the victim(s). Thus, preserving perhaps a few precious minutes of the "Golden Hour," for the trauma physician to work with. Remember, that Golden Hour started ticking away when the crash occurred, not when you arrived on the scene.

I am only going to give you one method for each task, nothing complicated and nothing fancy. It won't be anything that two trained persons cannot work to perfection and probably most important, it will be **affordable**.

The methods I have chosen are those which I have used many, many times and I know they work! You should not have to be kicked in the head to realize when you need help. But when help is a long time coming, these skills should go a long way toward stretching that magical hour.

Please pay particular attention to the Tool List. Though, not lengthy, it is imperative you purchase the best. This is not a place for broken tools.

Train, train, train! Be sure you know your tools and your limitations. There will be few times when you will not be ready to transport long before help arrives.

Good luck! If you have any questions, you know where I am.

– Jim Gargan

ACKNOWLEDGMENTS

Many hours have gone into this book, with the encouragement and help of a lot of people. At the risk of missing someone, I will endeavor to thank the following:

ROY L. ALSON, M.D. PH.D. - Assistant Professor, Department of Emergency Medicine, Bowman Gray School of Medicine, A special thank you to Dr. Alson for writing the material on emergency care procedures.

JERE BALDWIN, M.D. - Former Chairman of the Board, BTLS International.

JOHN A. CAMPBELL, M.D. - President, BTLS International

ROBERT A. FISHER - Fire Service Advisor/Instructor, Alberta Fire Training School, Vermilion, Alberta, Canada.

WALTER IDOL, EMT-P - Chief Flight Paramedic, UT Life Star, University of Tennessee Medical Center at Knoxville.

LOU JORDAN, PA. - Publisher, Emergency Training Associates, Union Bridge, MD.

KNOXVILLE VOLUNTEER RESCUE SQUAD - Knoxville, Tennessee.

LES LOUGHEED, EMT-P - Chief Flight Mechanic, UT Life Star, University of Tennessee Medical Center at Knoxville.

DONNA HASTINGS McGEADY - Coordinator, Life Support Training, Grant MacEwan Community College, Edmonton, Alberta, Canada.

WILLIAM BRUCE PATTERSON - ALS Programmer, Grant MacEwan Community College, Edmonton, Alberta, Canada.

CHARLES "BROTHER" W. SMITH, JR., EMT - Senior Instructor, Rescue Training Consultants, Saltville, Virginia.

BERNARD VAN TIGHEM - Fire Services Advisor/Instructor, Alberta Fire Training School, Vermilion, Alberta, Canada.

The staged photos were taken at the Knoxville Volunteer Rescue Squad in Knoxville, Tennessee.

Appearing in the photos are: **JOHN WHITED, WALTER IDOL, DAVID BRACE, ANGELA BOWEN, DAWN OGLE, HENRY NEWTON, BRYAN BRANCH, KAREN WELLS, DAVID SIKES, SCOTT POTTER, CLYDE ISNER & MICKEY REA.**

Photography was by **LES LOUGHEED**. Slide photos for the BTLS Access Course were taken by **ROY ALSON, M.D.**

For her excellence in putting it all together in the computer, my secretary, **DEANNA "DEE" BELAY.**

And finally, for putting up with it all, the lady who makes it all tick, my wife, **BARBARA.**

ABOUT THE AUTHOR

James B. Gargan is a resident of Kure Beach, North Carolina where he presides as the President of Rescue Training Consultants.

1995 marks Mr. Gargan's 47th anniversary in the emergency services. He served as Chief of the Prospect Park (PA) Fire Department and was active for many years as an instructor for the Pennsylvania State Fire School. He was Director of the Delaware County (PA) Fire School, teaching fire and rescue skills throughout eastern Pennsylvania.

Mr. Gargan is a member of the International Association of Fire Chiefs, serving on the Transportation Emergency Rescue Committee. He is a member of the Eastern Association of Fire Chiefs and the Delaware County (PA) Firemen's Association. Mr. Gargan also serves on the Advisory Council to the Urban Search and Rescue Task Force of the Congressional Fire Services Caucus in Washington, D.C.

Jim Gargan serves on the Allegheny County (PA) Emergency Delta Team. He has appeared on many national seminars and training programs, and has written numerous articles for emergency service magazines.

James B. Gargan is the author of Trench Rescue, and co-author of the second edition of Vehicle Rescue and the Action Guide for Emergency Service Personnel. He is the inventor of the JIMMI-JAK pneumatic/mechanical stabilization system. Mr. Gargan also has his own company, J & B Equipment Company, Inc., of Wilmington, Delaware.

THE TOOLS TO DO THE JOB

Let us talk about the tools needed to quickly and efficiently perform in any situation where victims are trapped. We must keep in mind the limitations of space and also holding the cost to where virtually any rescue squad or ambulance service organization can afford it.

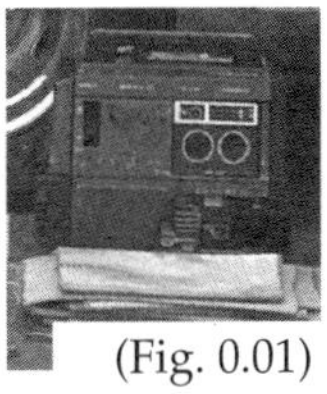

(Fig. 0.01)

The most expensive item will be a portable generator (Fig. 0.01). The main considerations here are weight, size and amperage rating. Examples, as provided by Honda, Generac, and Coleman, are but a few available. Fifteen amp output should be the smallest considered as this will allow the use of a tool and lighting. One twenty foot power cord with GFI (ground fault interrupter) built in, would be "Velcro-locked" to the end of the generator.

The only power tools in the system would be reciprocating saws. I would suggest both electric and gasoline powered saws. These are to be reinforced with at least ten short (4") and long (6") blades. This is no time to be thrifty. Be sure to buy the best blades available, such as Lenox Hackmaster 18 teeth per inch bi-metal blades.

I might also suggest a few extra long handled allen wrenches to fit the saws. Get rid of the trigger lock button. It can be dangerous to the inexperienced operator and serves no good purpose (Fig. 0.02).

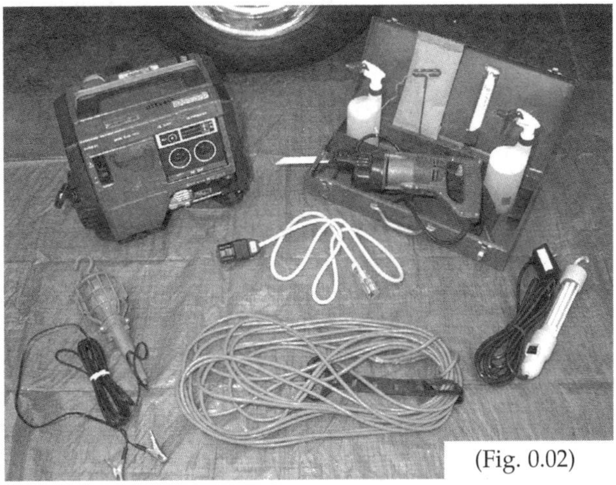

(Fig. 0.02)

Two single tube fluorescent work lights, one 12 volt with battery alligator clips, and one 120 volt should be carried for night work.

I also recommend a canvas masonry bag to hold all of the small hand tools (Fig. 0.03). It is lightweight and easily stored.

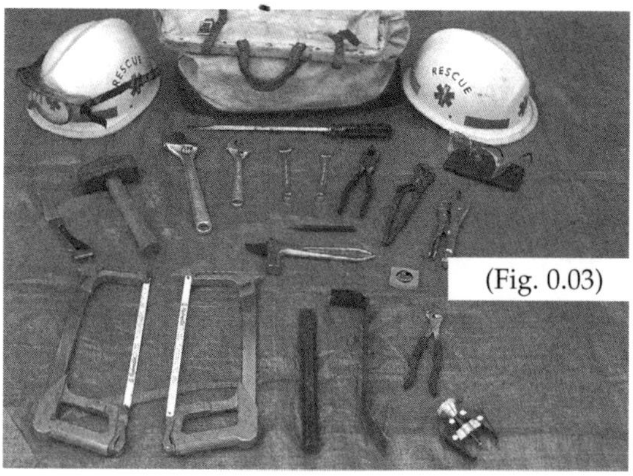

(Fig. 0.03)

Following is a list of equipment that should be stored in the bag:

2 — Rigid frame handheld hacksaws with at least ten spare blades, once again, Lenox Hackmaster 18 teeth per inch.
1 — 2 1/2 # machinists hammer
1 — 12″ Cold Chisel
1 — 16-inch large flat blade screwdriver
1 — Wonder bar (Stanley or Sears)
1 — Schild panel cutter
1 — Large side cutters
1 — Large (12″) crescent wrench
1 — Small (6″) crescent wrench
1 — 1/2″ combination open end and box wrench
1 — 14 mm Metric open end and box wrench
1 — 9/16″ combination open end and box wrench
1 — 15mm Metric open end and box wrench
1 — Center punch — spring loaded
1 — Large channel lock pliers
1 — Large vise grip pliers
1 — Heavy knife such as a buck knife
1 — Battery pliers
1 — Battery cable puller
1 — 8′ x 8′ lightweight tarpaulin
1 — Roll of duct tape
1 — Box of duct seal
2 — Squirt bottles with soapy water
12 — Golf tees
10 — Cyalume hi-intensity light sticks
1— 6′ retractable tape

Also carried are the following long tools:

1 — Quik-bar or Halligan Tool with pike
1 — 51″ Pinch bar
2 — Hi-Lift jacks

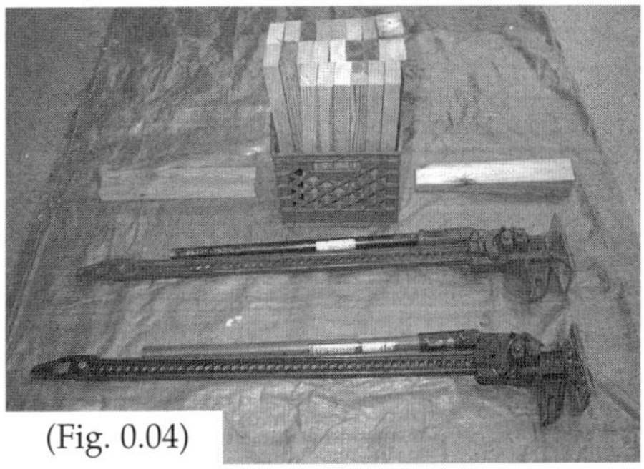

(Fig. 0.04)

If room permits, you might consider step cribs or a box of cribbing (Fig. 0.04). This would consist of a milk box with 21 pieces of 2″ x 4″ x 18″ cribbing with loops of lightweight rope stapled to the ends.

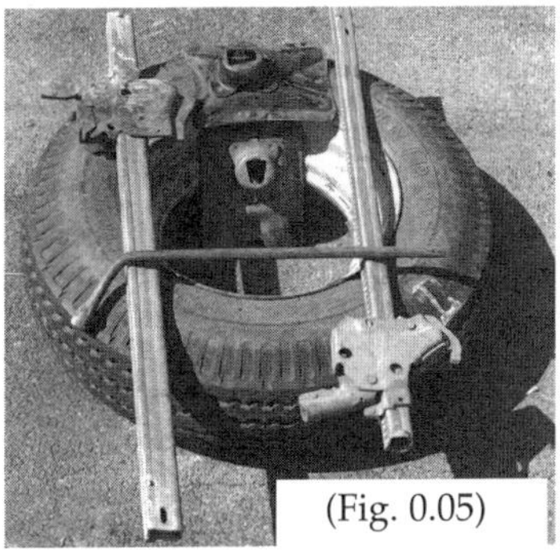

(Fig. 0.05)

On the scene you will be looking for: (Fig. 0.05).

— Spare tires
— Bumper jacks, both notch and con tour style
— Jack handles

The idea is to keep the tool kit at a minimum and yet be able to accomplish all of the tasks.

Rather than trying to impose a dress code, let me just say "appropriate" head, eye and hand protection should always be worn by all personnel performing the access procedures, (Fig. 0.06).

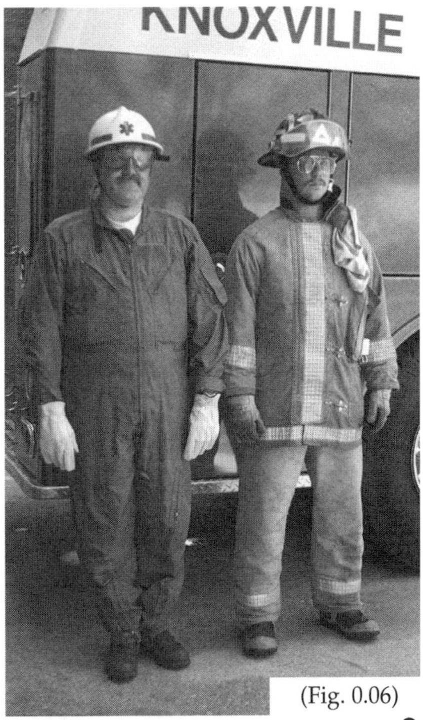

(Fig. 0.06)

Anatomy of an Automobile

Terminology You Should Know

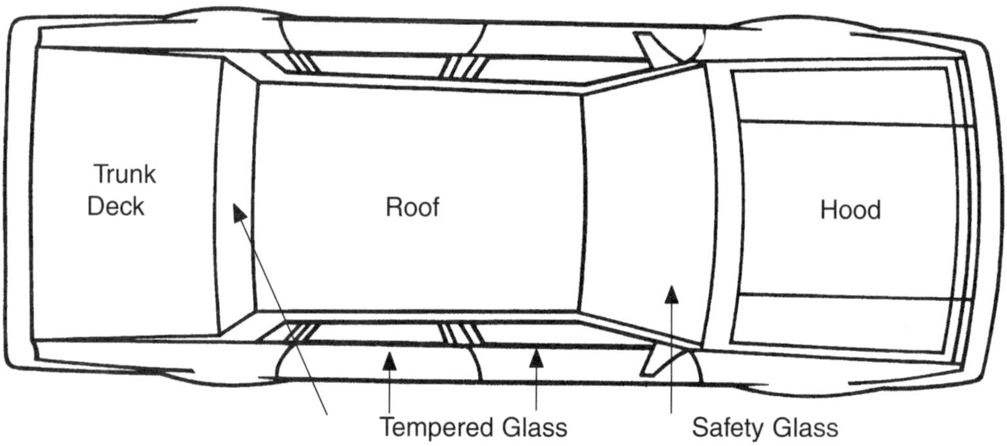

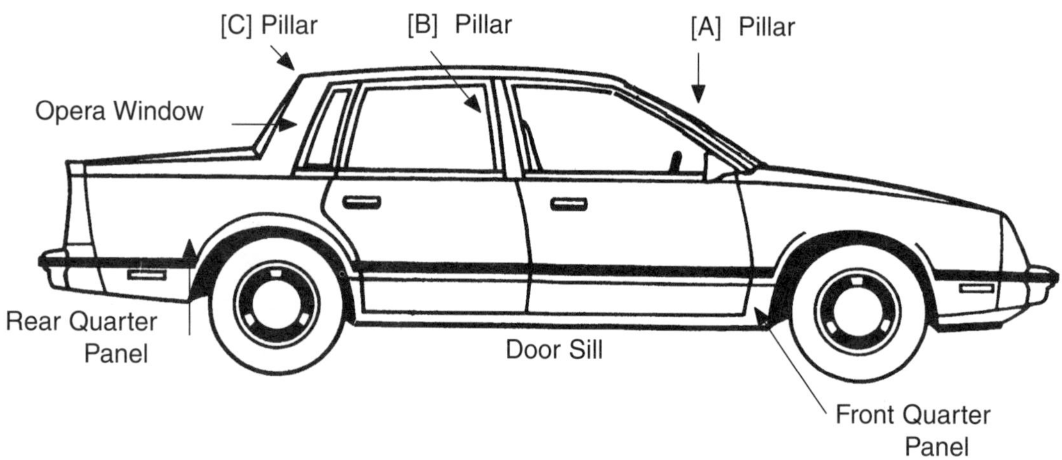

CHAPTER ONE

SIZE-UP

KNOWLEDGE OBJECTIVES

The rescuer should be able to...

- Summarize activities of the size-up phase;
- List at least 10 vehicle hazards that may be present at a vehicle accident;
- Recognize an unstable vehicle;
- Know when the situation is beyond his control;
- Know the operation of a supplemental restraint system;
- Determine the number of victims.

SKILL OBJECTIVES

The rescuer should be able to...

- Conduct a primary and secondary size up;
- Stop a minor gasoline leak;
- Disarm the supplemental restraint system;
- Triage the victims.

CHAPTER ONE

SIZE-UP

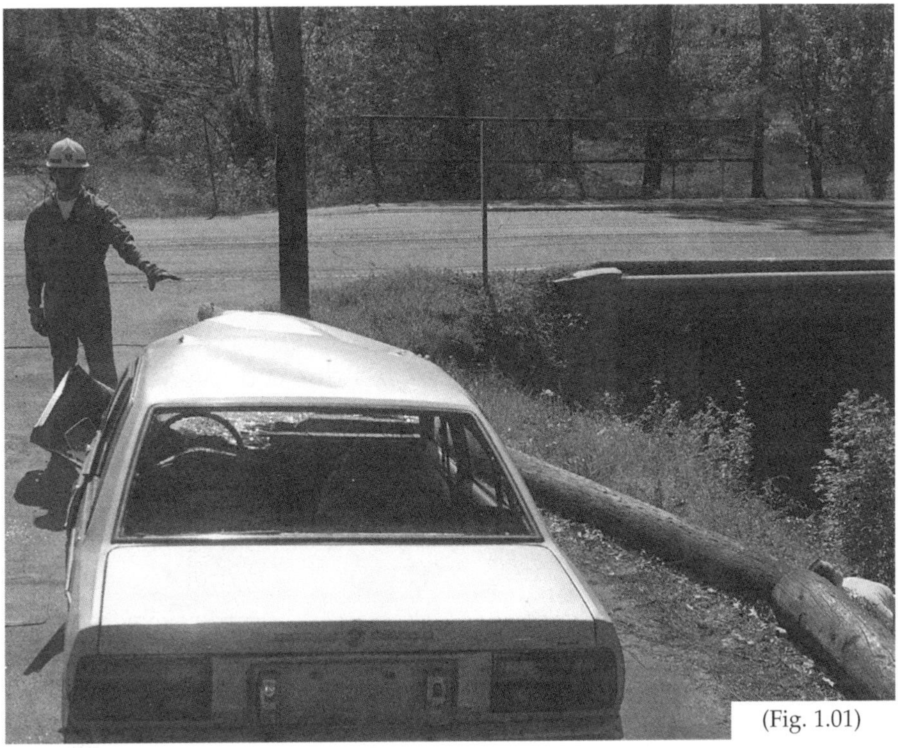

(Fig. 1.01)

Size-up, the overall assessment of the scene, must be done in a quick and concise manner.

You are looking for specifics to determine if you can do the job or not. When working with a single partner, you do not have a lot of time to formulate a plan as if you were setting up a command post. Yet, depending on the number of people and vehicles involved, that is exactly what you may end up doing.

By conducting a walk-around, you can quickly determine the number of victims both in and out of the vehicle(s), the severity of their injuries, and the hazards, if any, on or near the vehicle(s), (Fig. 1.01).

Did you locate the victim in the above photograph?

Always look inside, around, away from, and under the wrecked vehicle.

HAZARDS

Hazards abound at the scene of an accident. Most are caused by the accident, but some are natural and enhanced by the problem. Following are some of the more common hazards found at accident scenes.

Downed Wires

In many areas, EMT's and paramedics are not versed in handling downed wires. End of lesson! (Thou shalt not fry thy help.)

The only thing you can do is set-up warning devices (flares, lights, etc.) to avoid having someone else injured. Remember, downed power lines do not always go to ground thus tripping the circuit. They can remain very much alive and not arcing. Always look overhead upon arrival on the accident scene. You are looking for dangling wires (especially hard to see at night), a pole mounted transformer which may be loose if the vehicle struck the pole, and the pole itself if it snapped on impact.

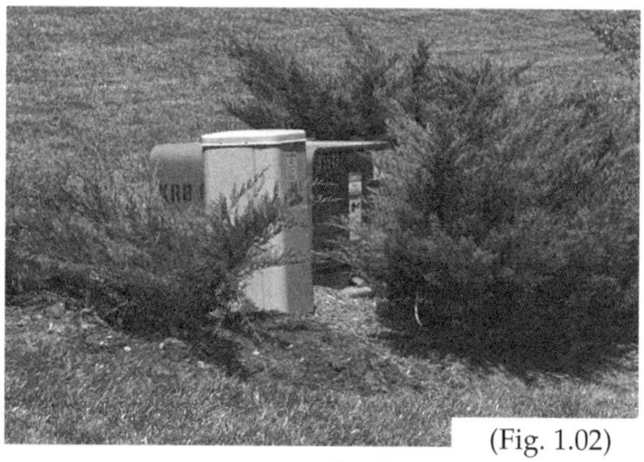

(Fig. 1.02)

Pad mounted transformers have become very popular as power lines are placed underground (Fig. 1.02). A vehicle can shear off a transformer and come to rest on top of it without cutting the power. This action is supposed to automatically shutdown the power, but nothing is for certain. On your size-up round, check under the vehicle(s).

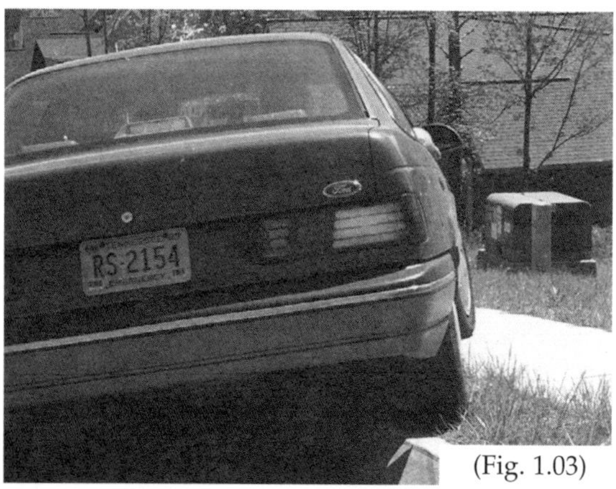

(Fig. 1.03)

Do not take a chance on touching the vehicle(s) if it is sitting on a transformer.

Immediately notify the power company if you are not equipped to handle the situation (Fig. 1.03).

Fuel Spill

If an accident vehicle has passed over debris or even a guardrail, chances are the fuel system has been damaged.

If the fuel tank has a gash in it of any size, it will have dumped before you arrive on the scene. Look for a pool of gasoline or diesel fuel during size up.

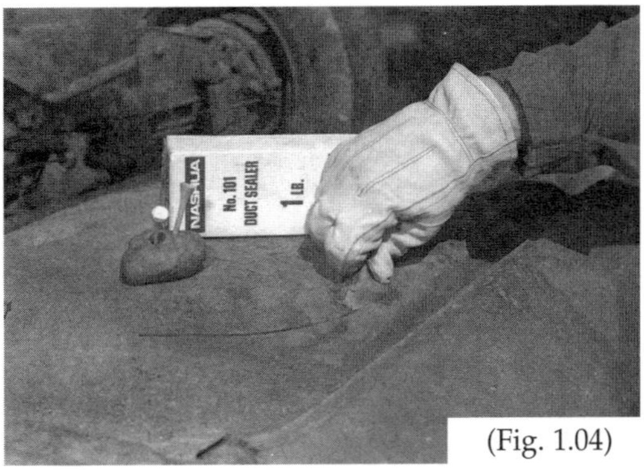

(Fig. 1.04)

If it is a minor leak, it can be stopped by pushing duct seal into the cut or puncture (Fig. 1.04).

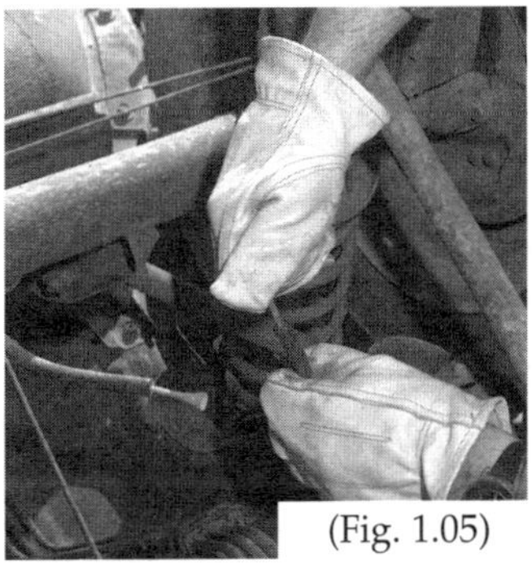
(Fig. 1.05)

If fuel lines are pulled loose, push a golf tee as far into the rubber line as possible (Fig. 1.05). Remember, if the key is still on, the electric fuel pump will continue to flow fuel if a line is broken.

Instability

A car that has been involved in an accident that has injured the occupant(s) must be considered unstable with regard to a possible C-spine injury or any other injury that can be aggravated by the movement of the vehicle.

Regardless of the position of the vehicle, all spring action or possible movement of the vehicle must be eliminated before the medic team goes to work on the victim(s). The safety of the rescuers is also a prime consideration. A chapter devoted to stabilization follows.

Natural Hazards

Curbs, swales, meter boxes, hydrants, and raised flower beds are all tripping hazards that, after dark, can put a halt to the operation by causing a sprained ankle. So be careful in your footing and always carry a light after nightfall.

Roadside drainage ditches present special problems when the vehicle rolls over and comes to rest upside down in the ditch. This action precludes entry through the doors. This situation will be discussed extensively in Chapter Four.

Creeks, rivers, lakes, ponds or any other body of water where the vehicle may end up submerged are beyond the scope of this book and will not be discussed. When confronted with this type of incident, make certain appropriate units are dispatched to the scene.

Air Restraint Bags

To even mention airbags in the presence of some people is to trip the trigger of gloom as to the many so called problems associated with them.

I might remind you the alternative in many cases is called death. Out of ignorance comes sanctimonious censure of probably the finest and most effective safety devise ever installed in our automobiles, if used with lap-shoulder belts. We could liken it to the hue and cry raised when shock absorbing bumpers were the whipping boy to those who would chain them or even drill them, when in fact, you need only know there could be a problem, so you work around them.

Knowing how the airbags operate is probably the key to being comfortable with them.

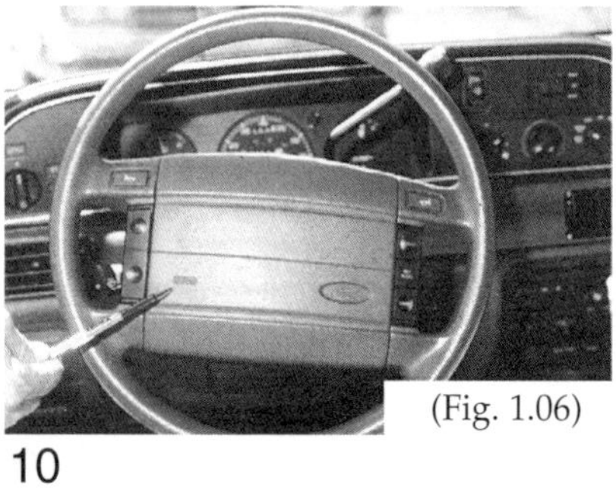

(Fig. 1.06)

The sudden stopping of a vehicle (in a range of 8-15 miles per hour or more) causes the forward movement of a sensor devise which electrically starts a burning reaction inside a hermetically sealed container, located in the center of the steering wheel (Fig. 1.06). This burning produces an inert gas (nitrogen) which in turn fills the bag (s), thus halting the forward progress of the driver and passenger, if the lap-shoulder belts are in place. All of this in less time than it takes to blink (1/4 th of a second).

The bag(s) deflate immediately. Any powder residue seen will have been placed in the packaging of the bag by the manufacturer, as an anti-sticking substance. Talcum powder and cornstarch are two of the mediums commonly used.

Minute particles of a slightly alkaline powder may be present as a by-product of the sodium azide used to produce the gas. This could cause a minor caustic burn or allergic reaction.

Recent studies show cervical fractures, apparently from hyperextention, showing up in some airbag deployment accidents. Most of the injuries were with drivers who were not restrained by lap-shoulder belts.

If the air bag does not deploy, as in a side or rear collision, simply disarm the system by disconnecting the negative (black) cable on the vehicle's battery. The capacitors used to fire the system will drain off quickly. Do not delay the rescue/treatment effort, just work around the bag area. Chances of an accidental deployment are nil.

ACCIDENT VICTIMS

Identifying the number of victims from an accident is one of the most important functions of your size-up. A good survey of the scene will show how many persons are supposed to be in the vehicle(s). Note the words "supposed to be." Victims could be ejected in a roll-over, trauma victims may walk away from the scene, or the wreckage could be hiding the victim.

If no one is conscious on your arrival, try to fix the numbers of victims by looking for clues such as schoolbooks and/or lunch pails but no children, three briefcases and top coats, but only two men in the car. Look for things of this nature that do not add up. Be suspicious.

This is triage time! And though the DUI pinned behind the wheel is bleeding profusely and wailing like a baby, his cuts may be superficial. Beware of the non—speaking person staring straight ahead and saying nothing. Triage your patients based upon your BTLS primary survey.

KEY POINTS TO REMEMBER

- Specifics of vehicle design will vary between car manufacturers, such as:

  Location of the fuel tank
  Type of fuel pump-mechanical vs. electric
  Door latch mechanisms
  Hinges - cast vs. pressed
  Location of batteries
  Uni-body vs. frame

  It is important to familiarize yourself with the basics of vehicle design

- Do not use "Silly Putty", modeling clay, or any petroleum based product that will dissolve in gasoline.

- Supplemental Restraint Systems (Airbags):

  Powder on surface of the airbag(s) is either talc or cornstarch. It is harmless.
  The amount of sodium azide in the sealed canister is only 90 grams. It cannot leak out.
  During deployment, the sodium azide is consumed.
  Inflation is to a pressure of 4 P.S.I.

- Hazard control is extremely important:

  Be aware of your surroundings.
  Do not assume someone else is going to correct the problem.
  Always think of downed wires as LIVE!
  Look up, around and under the vehicle.
  Roadside ditches can be "highways" for wildlife such as snakes and alligators.
  Immersion in water increases the risk of hypothermia in both victims and rescuers.
  Flowing water exerts tremendous force. It can easily sweep away victims and rescuers.

Unless completely familiar with the scene, never wade in water unless tethered to a lifeline.
Victims can be anywhere:
If victim is conscious, ask if anyone else is involved.
Look for clues that victim may have wandered off-foot prints in snow or mud, crushed weeds or broken branches.
Check glove compartment for victim's identification

NOTES:

JOTTING DOWN IMPORTANT INFORMATION WILL HELP YOU REMEMBER AND EXPAND YOUR KNOWLEDGE

SPACE FOR NOTES IS PROVIDED AFTER EACH CHAPTER FOR YOU TO ADD YOUR OWN "BITS AND PIECES" OF INFORMATION.

NOTES:

CHAPTER TWO

CALL FOR HELP AND SET UP

KNOWLEDGE OBJECTIVES:
The rescuer should be able to...

- **Determine the exact location of the accident scene;**

- **List the tools needed to accomplish the rescue;**

- **Know and describe where to place the tools.**

SKILL OBJECTIVES:
The rescuer should be able to...

- **Report the exact location of the accident scene;**

- **Set up the equipment needed;**

- **Gather additional devices needed for stabilization.**

CHAPTER TWO

CALL FOR HELP AND SET UP

Call For Help

Barring any unforeseen circumstances, the size-up should only take seconds rather than minutes. Upon returning to your vehicle if you are not equipped with portable radios, your next communication with your dispatcher should be considered your last before extrication of the victim. The most important message is your final and exact location.

A brief summation of the number of victims and their entrapment problems along with requests for support equipment would be about the extent of your message. Remember, you have not yet stabilized the vehicle(s), so you have not gotten to the primary survey yet.

If you have portable communications, then you will be able to give a blow by blow account of the situation later.

Setting up the equipment is next.

Setting up

Spread the tarp on the ground placing the generator on one corner, Quik Bar on another corner, Hi-Lift Jack on another, etc., so as to secure the tarp from blowing with the wind.

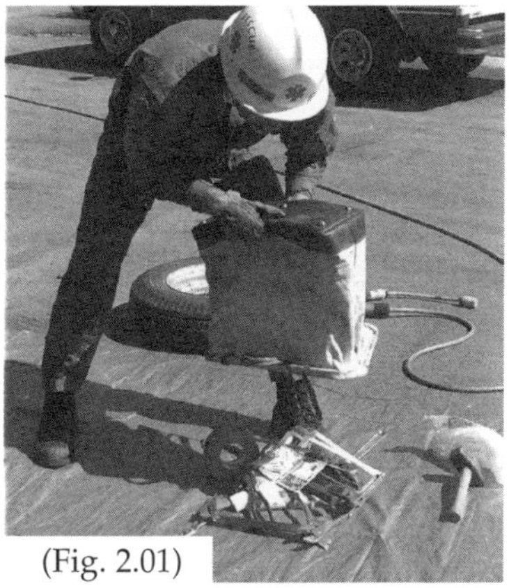

(Fig. 2.01)

Dump the contents of the canvas bag discussed earlier directly in the center of the tarp (Fig. 2.01).

It is much easier to see the tool of choice this way, rather than groping in the bag for it, and much safer and less painful than blindly reaching in the bag and getting stuck or cut by a sharp tool (Fig. 2.02).

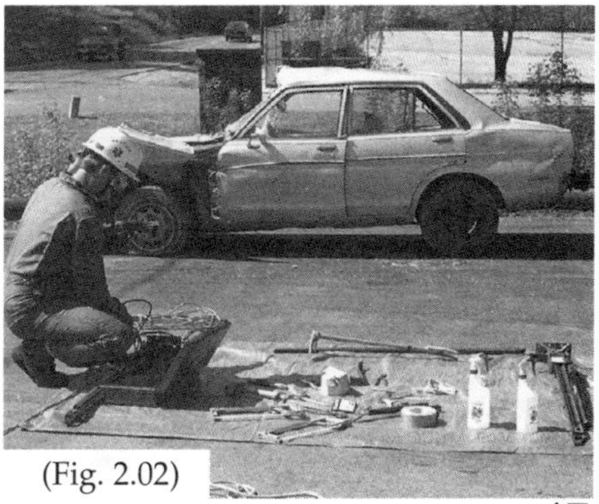

(Fig. 2.02)

This action should be done within ten feet of the side of the vehicle to be entered. Allow enough room to remove doors or drop the side without setting up a tripping hazard.

All tools must be returned to the tarp after use to avoid losing them in grass or having them kicked under debris or the vehicle. Long tools, cribbing or any tools not being used should be on the tarp at all times.

Depending upon stabilization needs, while one medic is setting up the tool depot, his partner could be gathering stabilization devices such as bumper jacks (both notch style and contour style), jack handles, scissor jacks, hub caps and spare tires. These could be from the victim's car, passersby cars, police cars or even the ambulance.

KEY POINTS TO REMEMBER

- **Call for help should include:**

  Number of victims.
  Condition of victims.
  Exact location of the call.
  Specific hazards.
  Additional help needed for patient care and hazards.
  Safe route to the scene.

NOTES:

JOTTING DOWN IMPORTANT INFORMATION WILL HELP YOU REMEMBER AND EXPAND YOUR KNOWLEDGE

SPACE FOR NOTES IS PROVIDED AFTER EACH CHAPTER FOR YOU TO ADD YOUR OWN "BITS AND PIECES" OF INFORMATION.

NOTES:

CHAPTER THREE

STABILIZATION

KNOWLEDGE OBJECTIVES:
The rescuer should be able to...

- **List the positions in which a vehicle is unstable.**

SKILL OBJECTIVES:
The rescuer should be able to...

- **Stabilize a vehicle on its wheels;**
- **Stabilize a vehicle on its roof edge;**
- **Stabilize a vehicle on its tire edge;**
- **Stabilize a vehicle on its roof;**
- **Stabilize a vehicle with spare tires only.**

CHAPTER THREE

STABILIZATION

Stabilization is as critical to the victim as proper packaging. The art of rendering a wrecked vehicle motionless is as important as putting a collar on an accident victim.

Why? Because the medic cannot guarantee the vehicle will not roll over or be still long enough to fit a collar. How many quadriplegics or paraplegics have we created by sloppy work in an unstable vehicle?

When properly stabilized, the vehicle should have no appreciable movement. This can be accomplished in as little as fifteen seconds, so there is no excuse to work in an unsafe, unstable vehicle, jeopardizing both the victim and the rescuers.

I will address every manner in which a vehicle can be unstable along with the method used to stabilize. This includes: a car on its wheels, a car on its roof edge (side up), a car on it's tire edge (side up), and a car on its roof.

Car on Its Wheels

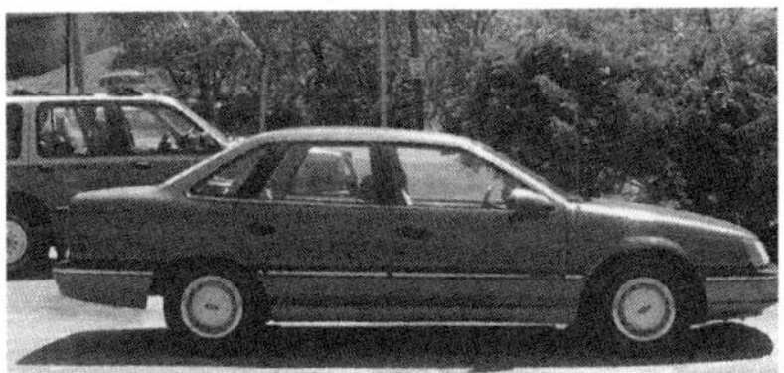

(Fig.3.01)

Certainly the most common of unstable vehicles are those found still on their wheels (Fig. 3.01).

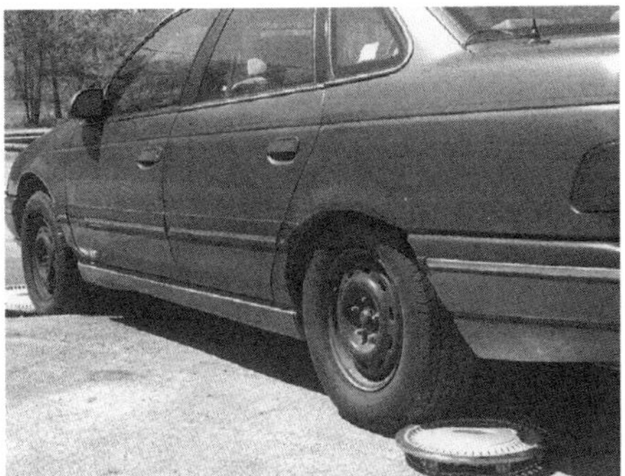

(Fig. 3.02)

The first consideration is to chock the car in the position found by popping the hub caps and placing them in front of the front wheel and to the rear of the rear wheel (Fig. 3.02).

If the hub caps are of the locking type, use the wheel chocks (Fig. 3.03), from the emergency vehicle or a few pieces of cribbing (Fig. 3.04).

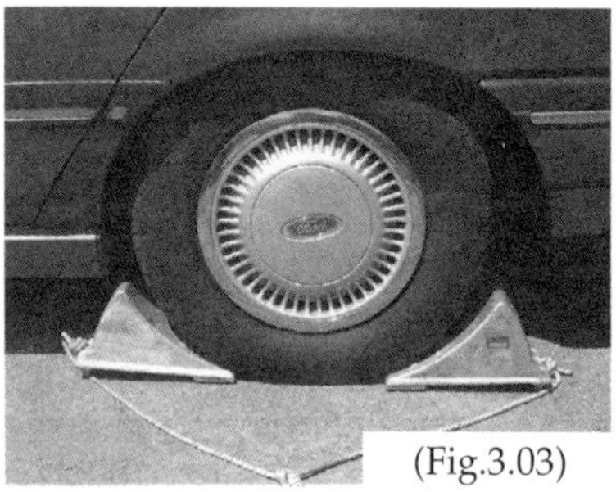
(Fig.3.03)

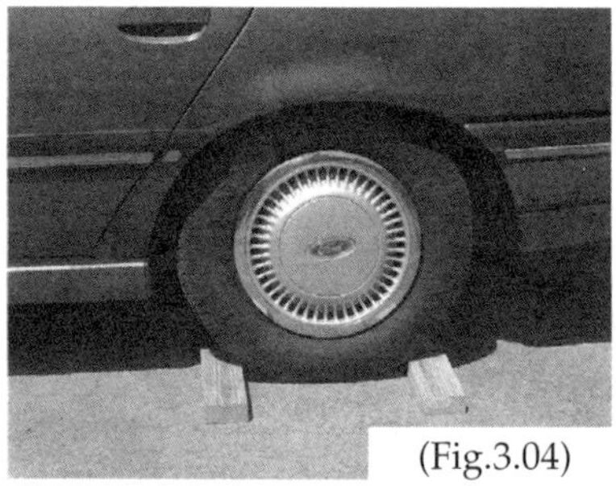
(Fig.3.04)

The key is preventing the vehicle from moving, even uphill. Never assume the car will not move even when a flat tire is evident.

The next step is to build box cribs under the "A" pillars and ahead of the rear wheels (Fig. 3.05). Place your back against the wheel well and lift the side of the car, taking the spring action out of the body as your partner slides the cribbing in place.

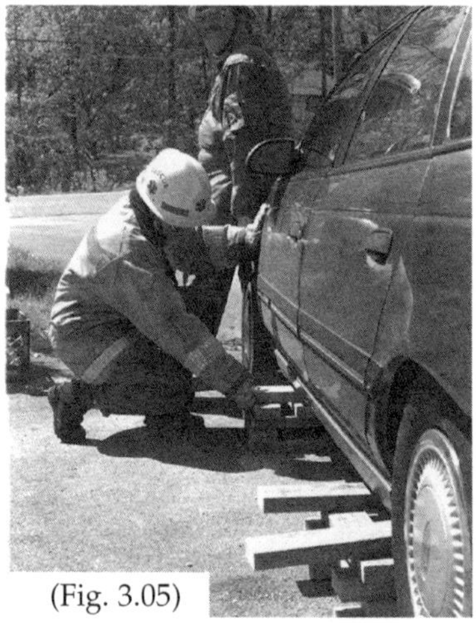
(Fig. 3.05)

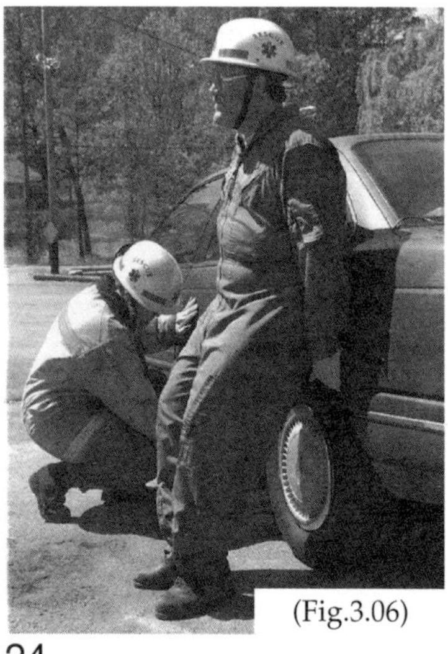
(Fig.3.06)

Repeat this procedure for the rear wheel and then the other side (Fig. 3.06). Always lift with your legs, not your back.

With the vehicle setting on cribbing, take the side cutters from the tool kit and walk around the car pulling the valve stems (Fig. 3.07). As the suspension system relaxes, it will tighten up the car on the cribbing.

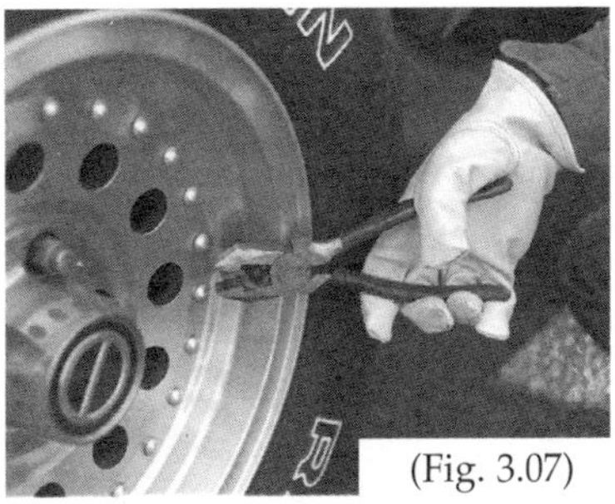
(Fig. 3.07)

Car on Its Side — Resting on the Roof Edge

Most cars will balance on the roof edge or drip mold, with the wheels not touching the ground (Fig. 3.08). This is perhaps the most dangerous position as the car could roll on you or continue on over onto the roof when touched, thus causing tragic results to those inside the vehicle.

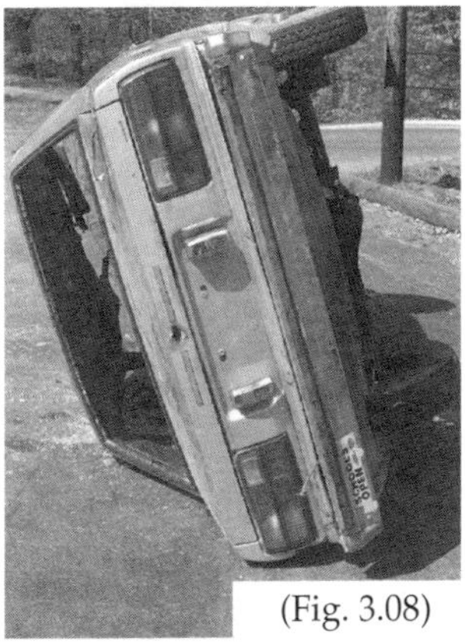
(Fig. 3.08)

To stabilize a vehicle in this position, you will want to plan ahead to determine how you will remove the victim(s). The easiest method is to cut the roof on one side and lay it down.

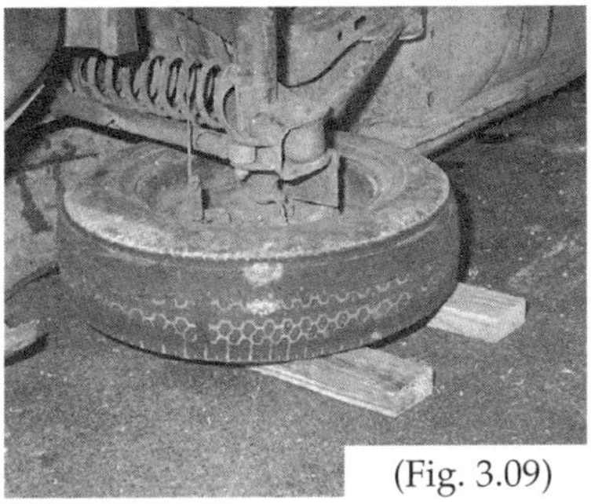
(Fig. 3.09)

Start by building a box crib and sliding it under the rear wheel (Fig. 3.09).

Position your partner and yourself at opposite ends of the vehicle and gently push the car onto the cribbing (Fig. 3.10).

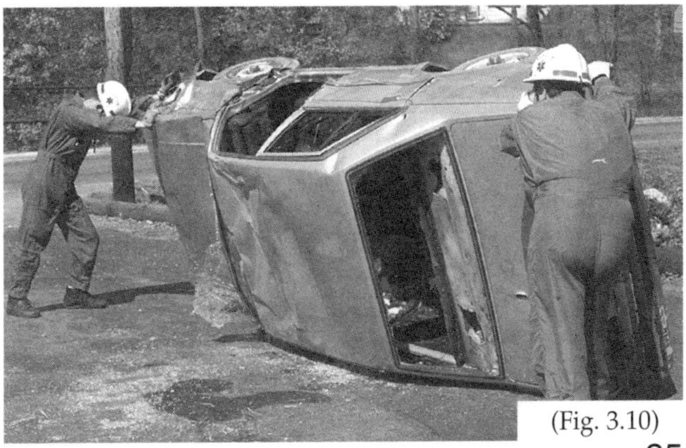
(Fig. 3.10)

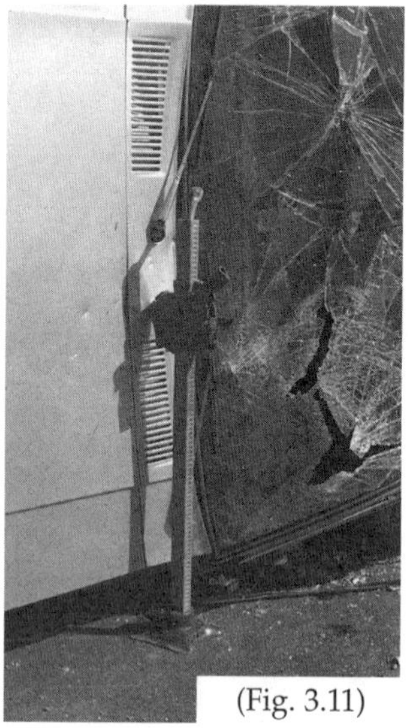

(Fig. 3.11)

The cribbing should be centered on the wheel rather than the tire. As your partner holds the vehicle in place by pushing on the roof, use the Quik Bar to make a hole in the cowling behind the hood (in front of the windshield), and rotate the Quik Bar to a vertical position pulling down on it gently. You will thus corrugate the hole and make easy access to the notch-style bumper jack. Place the jack on the ground beneath the hole and insert the blade (Fig. 3.11). Jack only until tight. Do not lift the vehicle.

The bumper jack or the Hi-Lift Jack could also be placed into the trunk deck (Fig. 3.12, 3.13, and 3.14).

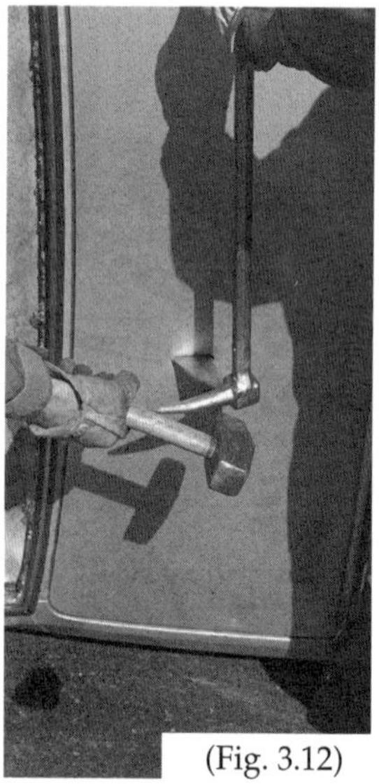

(Fig. 3.12)

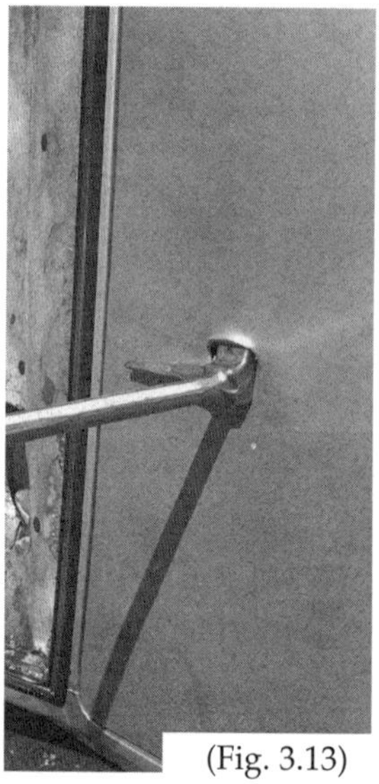

(Fig. 3.13)

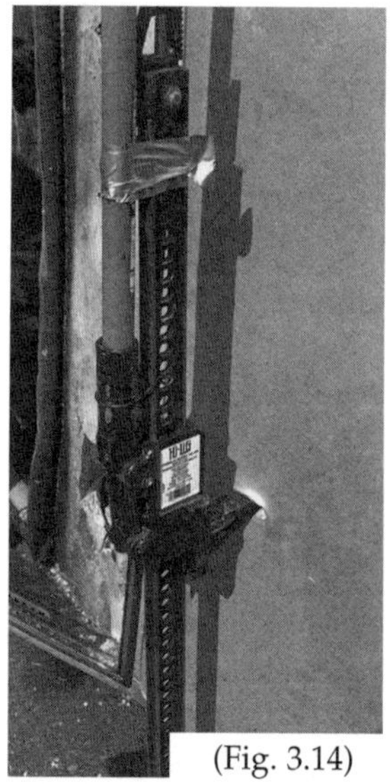

(Fig. 3.14)

In this case, the cribbing would go under the front wheel (Fig. 3.15).

Always crib and stabilize on a diagonal; never directly across from each other, thus setting up a pivot point on which the car will rotate.

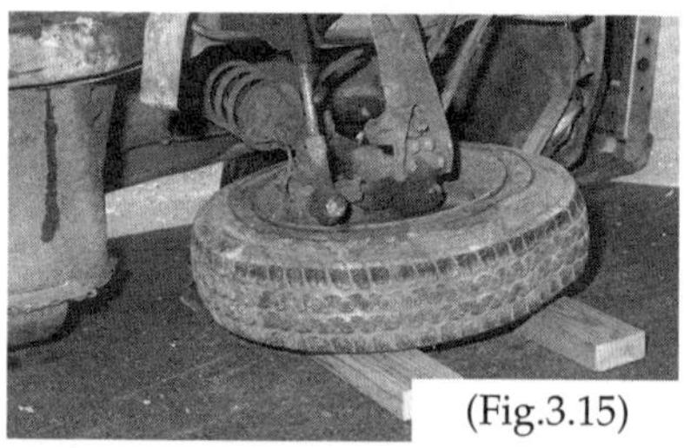

(Fig.3.15)

Car on Its Side — Resting on Tire Edge

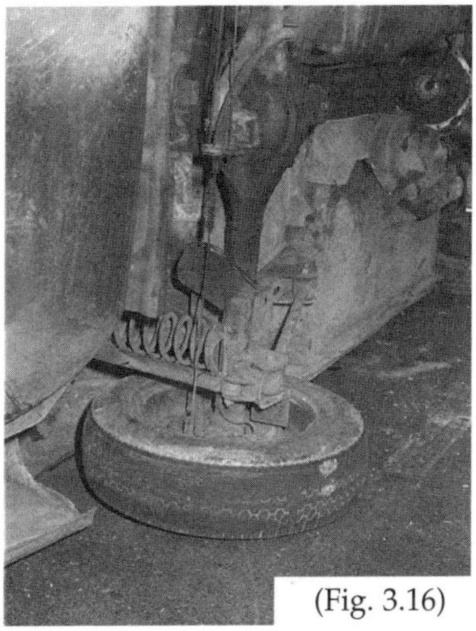

(Fig. 3.16)

Virtually the same situation but more stable (Fig. 3.16). The ideal situation would be to move the vehicle into a 90° position by again placing cribbing under the rear wheel. However, the weight of most cars will preclude this method. Instead, we will stabilize the vehicle as we find it. Use the Quik Bar to make the opening and the bumper jack in either the front cowling or trunk deck. If a bumper jack is not available, you can make a larger opening and use a Hi-Lift Jack. Again, it is vitally important that you not lift the car.

Car on Its Roof

Normally a car on its roof will come to rest with it's nose down because of the engine weight. However, some will balance on the roof. This presents real stability problems as the vehicle wants to rotate. If this is the case, place the spare tire under the center of the hood front (Fig. 3.17).

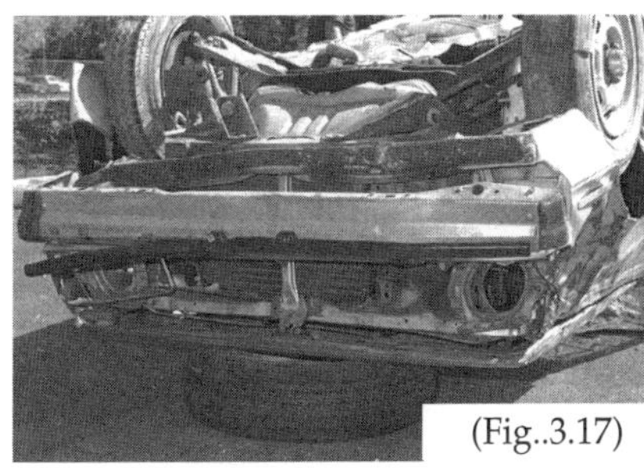

(Fig..3.17)

First make openings in the "C" pillars (Fig. 3.18, 3.19).

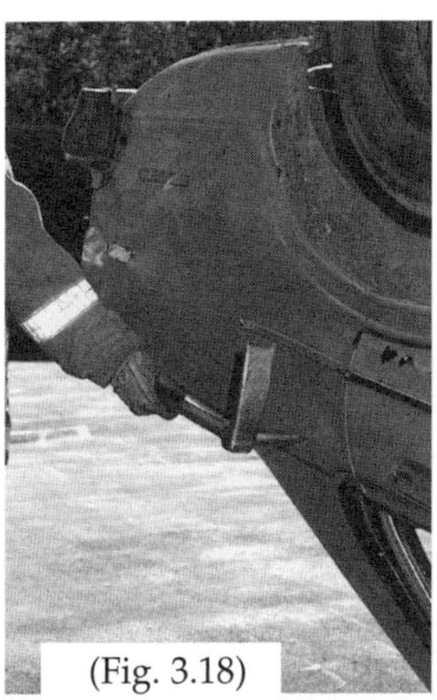

(Fig. 3.18)

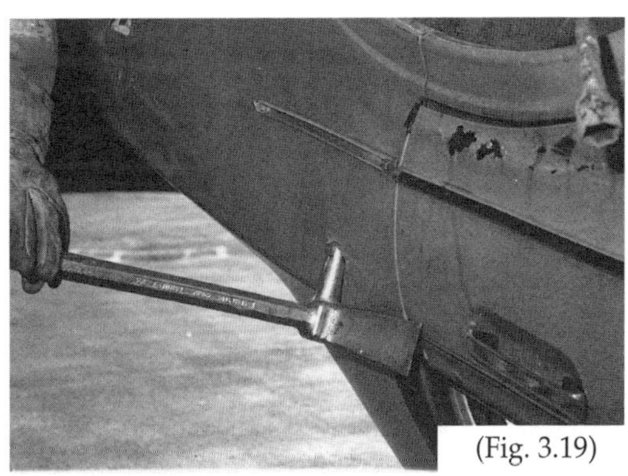

(Fig. 3.19)

Next, jack the car onto the tire until it is tight , 3.20 and 3.21).

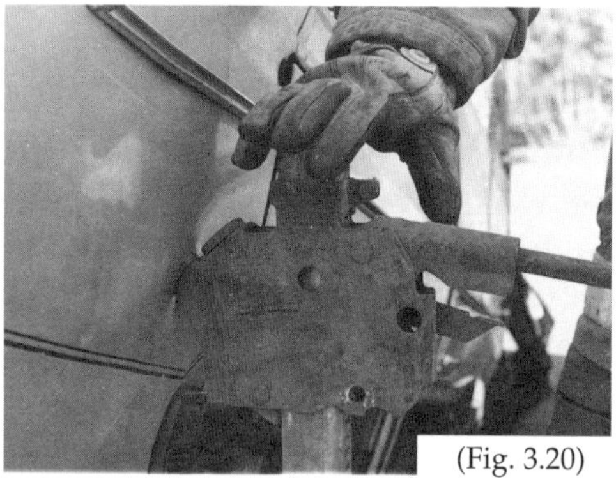

(Fig. 3.20)

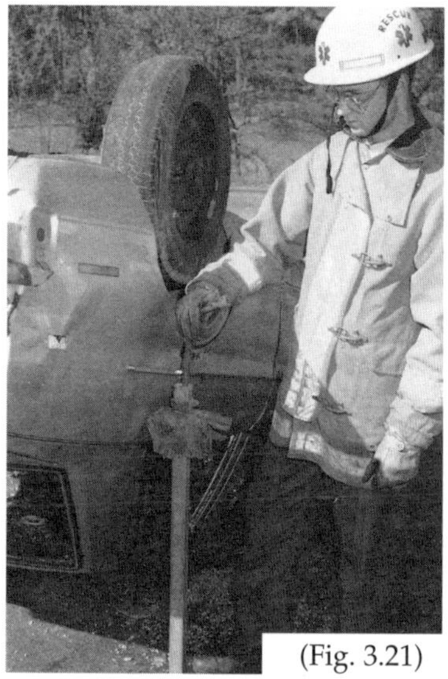

(Fig. 3.21)

Vehicles equipped with opera windows or slit glass adapt very well to this method as you only have to break the glass to insert the jacks (Fig. 3.22).

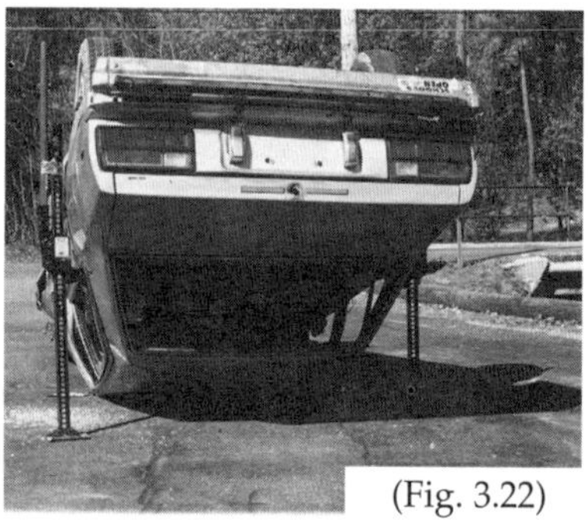

(Fig. 3.22)

You can also crib the rear of the roof at the rear window (Fig. 3.23).

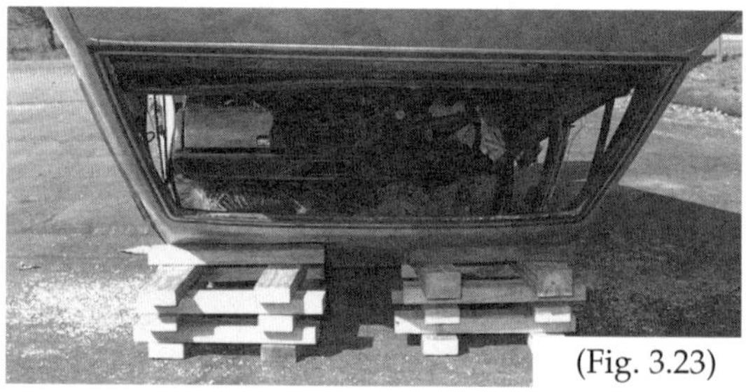

(Fig. 3.23)

Using Spare Tires

Most vehicles can be stabilized by using spare tires only, as long as they are the appropriate size. In the case of the vehicle on its wheels, simply place the spare tires under the "A" pillars on each side and pull the valve stems on all four tires of the vehicle (Fig. 3.24).

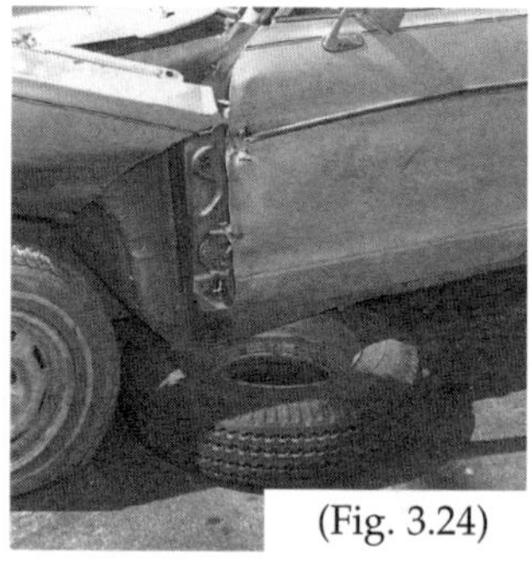

(Fig. 3.24)

With the cars on their sides, a spare tire under the rear wheel of the car on its roof edge and one under the "A" pillar will suffice.

The car on its tire edge needs only a spare tire under the "A" pillar (Fig. 3.25).

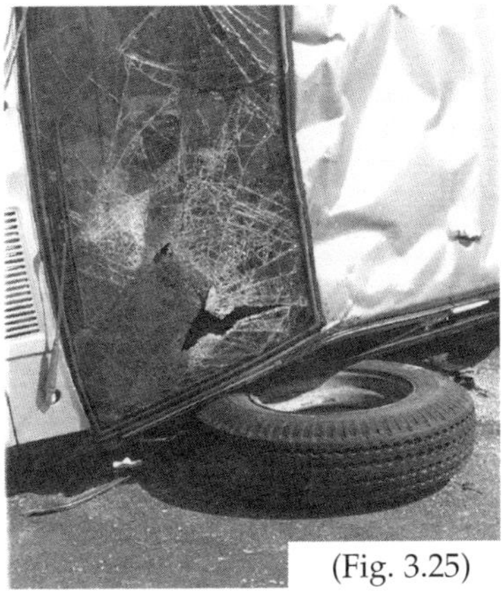
(Fig. 3.25)

You must remember by using spare tires, you will not get as rigid a job as with the other methods, because you will have inflated rubber which has much more "give" to it.

However, you are not compromising safety to the medics because the spare tires by themselves give you a much broader base.

There are many ways to stabilize a vehicle. I chose these few to avoid confusion and for their simplicity. Remember, don't try to re-invent the wheel, just do it!

KEY POINTS TO REMEMBER

- **Do not puncture tires to flatten**
- **<u>NEVER</u> return car to upright position with victim inside**
- **When using jack, stabilize only, <u>DO NOT LIFT</u>!**
- **For safety and to avoid accidental release, secure handle of Hi-Lift jack in upright position and place bumper jack handle in center of shaft.**

NOTES:

JOTTING DOWN IMPORTANT INFORMATION WILL HELP YOU REMEMBER AND EXPAND YOUR KNOWLEDGE

SPACE FOR NOTES IS PROVIDED AFTER EACH CHAPTER FOR YOU TO ADD YOUR OWN "BITS AND PIECES" OF INFORMATION.

CHAPTER FOUR

ACCESSING

KNOWLEDGE OBJECTIVES:
The rescuer should be able to...

- Determine an access point in a vehicle;
- Describe the different types of glass in a vehicle;
- Describe procedures for safely breaking safety glass;
- Describe procedures for safely breaking tempered glass;
- List the tools used for the above skills;
- List the mechanics of securing a door;
- Describe the "crash zones" of vehicles;
- List the steps in opening doors;
- Describe the different hinges;
- Describe unbolting doors;
- Determine when a roof should be removed;
- Describe the sequence for removing a roof back to front;
- Describe the sequence for dropping a roof from a vehicle on its side;
- Describe removing the floor assembly from a vehicle;
- List the problems and solutions of an engine compartment fire;
- List the problems and solutions of a trunk compartment fire.

SKILL OBJECTIVES
The rescuer should be able to...

- Safely break safety glass;
- Safely break tempered glass;
- Open a door conventionally;
- Expose and cut the "nader" bolt;
- Expose and cut the hinges on doors;
- Remove doors;
- Unbolt doors;
- Remove a roof from back to front;
- Drop a roof from a vehicle on its side;
- Remove the floor assembly of a vehicle;
- Extinguish an engine compartment fire;
- Extinguish a trunk compartment fire.

CHAPTER FOUR

ACCESSING

Remember: No accessing of patients is done until the vehicle is stabilized.

WINDOWS

While gaining access into a vehicle through a window can be done rather quickly, it should be regarded as a "starter" place. Certainly we do not want to drag a victim through a window unless it is a last resort. In our discussion on windows, we will only address two types: safety glass and tempered glass.

Safety Glass

Safety glass is a composition glass molded like a sandwich and consists of a layer of butazite between two layers of glass (Fig. 4.01).

The butazite acts as a stiffener and as the glass is formed under high heat and pressure, it adheres itself to the plate glass.

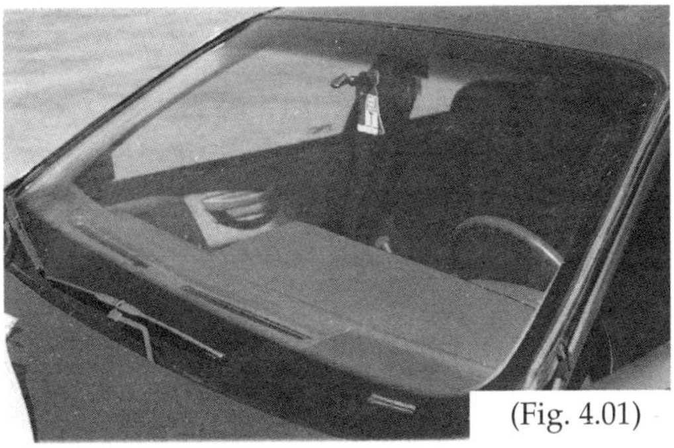

(Fig. 4.01)

Safety glass will crack rather easily but will not come apart. Thus, for the most part, safety glass will keep the occupants inside the vehicle even after taking a severe blow.

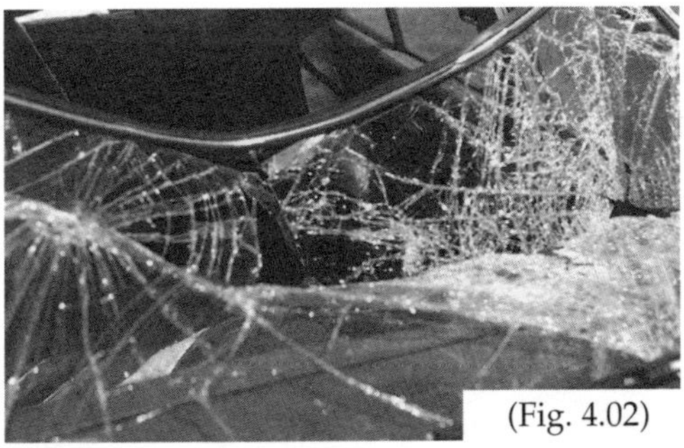

(Fig. 4.02)

Safety glass can be a double edged sword for medics, as the glass can pull off in large shards and cut quite severely as well as dust open wounds with a fine glass powder (Fig. 4.02). Any time you must go through glass, make sure the victim is completely covered.

At one time we would have used a windshield knife to completely remove the glass. Since the early eighties, the vehicle manufacturers have changed the mastic used to hold in the glass, thus, virtually eliminating the use of the knife. I would recommend the use of a saw or even an axe to remove safety glass (Fig. 4.03 and 4.04).

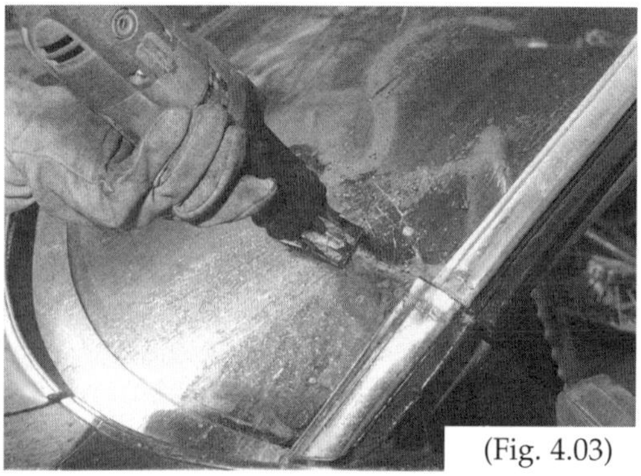

(Fig. 4.03)

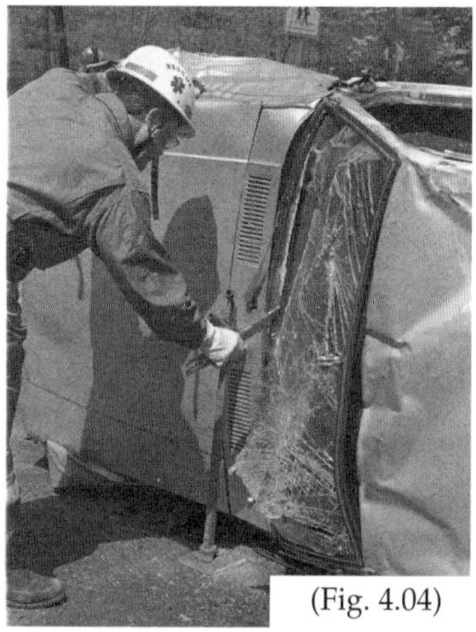

(Fig. 4.04)

Tempered Glass

Tempered glass will account for the rest of the windows in automobiles. This glass is also formed under high heat and pressure into a tough sheet without lamination and has a terrific memory (Fig. 4.05). It will bend and return without cracking. You may hit it with a heavy hammer and it will not break. But if you touch it with a sharp point, it will shatter into thousands of quarter-inch shards. Make no mistake, this glass will cut severely, but it will not normally produce the powder associated with safety glass.

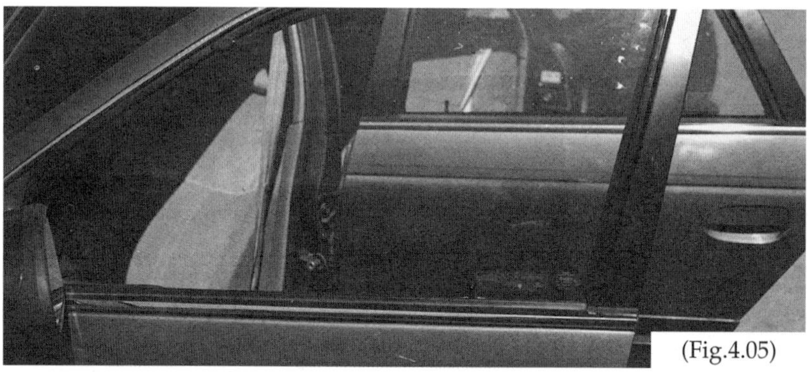

(Fig.4.05)

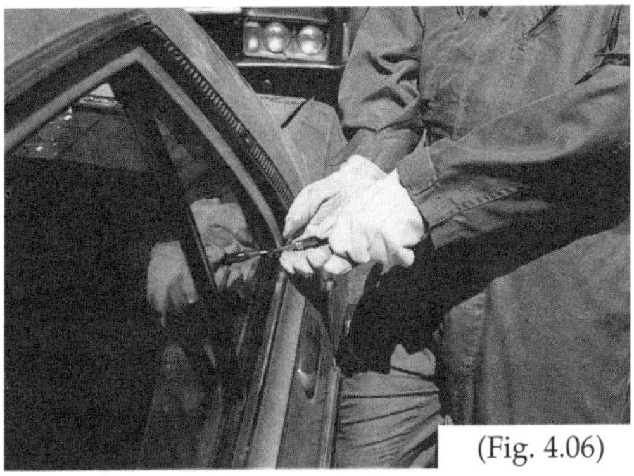

(Fig. 4.06)

The best means of access through tempered glass is the use of a spring loaded center punch placed in a lower corner of the window (Fig. 4.06).

Push gently and resist any forward motion of the hand or "follow thru;" this will shatter the glass (Fig. 4.07).

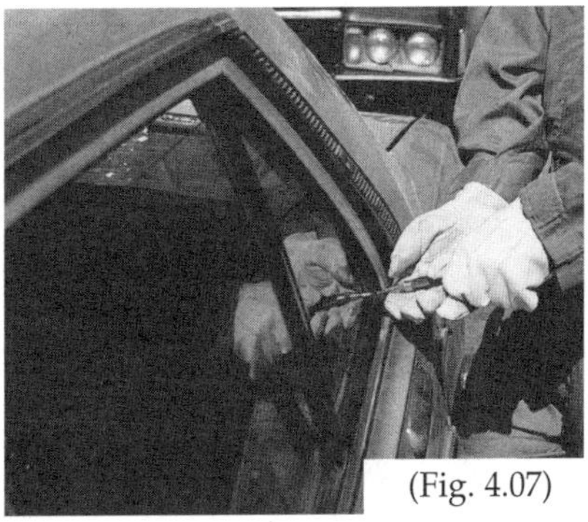

(Fig. 4.07)

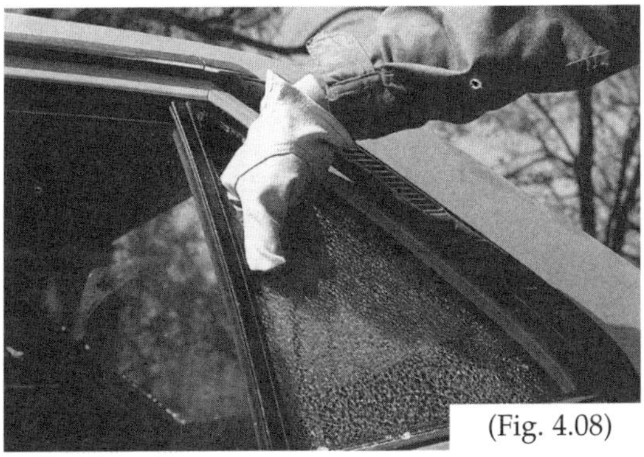

(Fig. 4.08)

Tap a few shards into the vehicle away from the victim, opening up a hand hole (Fig. 4.08). Reach in and pull all the glass to the outside.

A few other striking objects that can be used to shatter tempered glass are: a long, flat blade screwdriver, the flat blade end of a lug wrench (Fig. 4.09), a car aerial, and an engine dip stick. All of these are used in a whipping action.

When shattering glass, always work away from the victim if possible. Completely clean the entire opening of glass before proceeding.

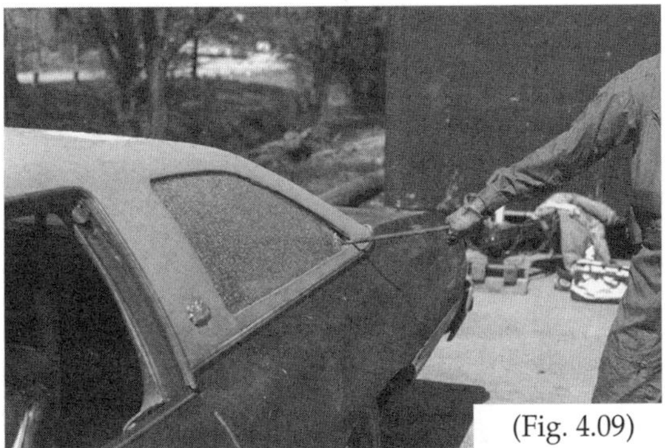

(Fig. 4.09)

DOORS

Doors can give you fits and make fools out of the best. For some reason, we forget the mechanics of securing a door. There are three: closing, latching and locking.

Before making any forcible entry through the windows or doors, try the latch! Surprise, it is open! Remember, a lot of thought has gone into developing "crash zones" into vehicles over the past few years. Vehicles will fold at preconceived points and most doors will operate even after a head-on collision. It is the "T-Bone" collision and rollover that cause real problems with doors.

The first step is to unlock the door. This can be accomplished by working the manual lock (up, on the mushroom head, or in direction shown on slide locks). Now it is a matter of unlatching.

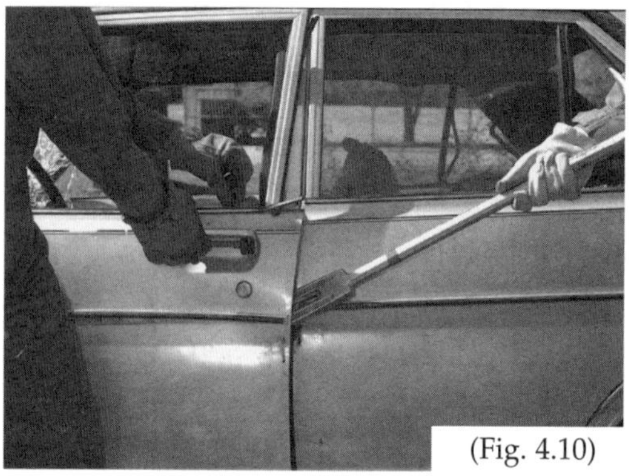

(Fig. 4.10)

If the door is jammed, try operating the unlatching handle or button, while your partner uses the halligan tool or pinch bar to force the door past the jam (Fig. 4.10).

The latch/lock box is a very sophisticated assembly. If the scissors of the latch (Fig. 4.11) are jammed around the lock pin (Naider bolt) (Fig. 4.12), you are not about to break it.

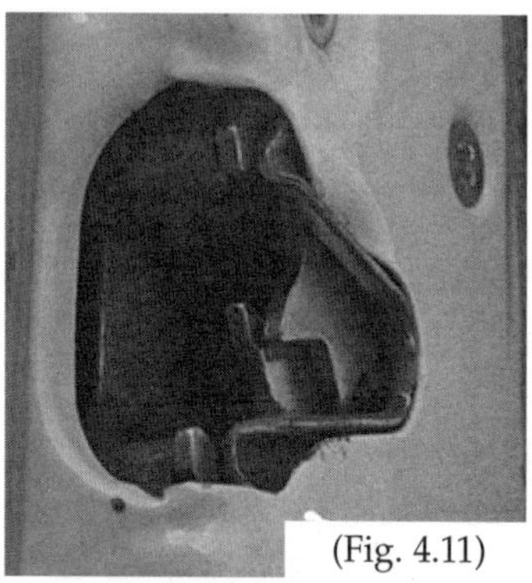

(Fig. 4.11)

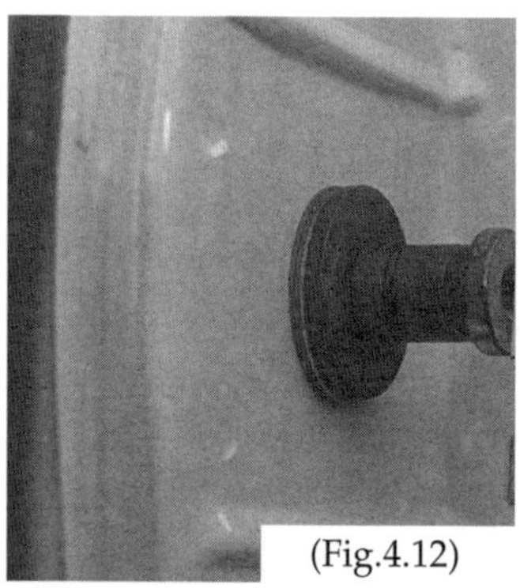

(Fig.4.12)

Two methods can be used. With the halligan tool, bend the lip of the door back to expose the lock bolt (Fig. 4.13).

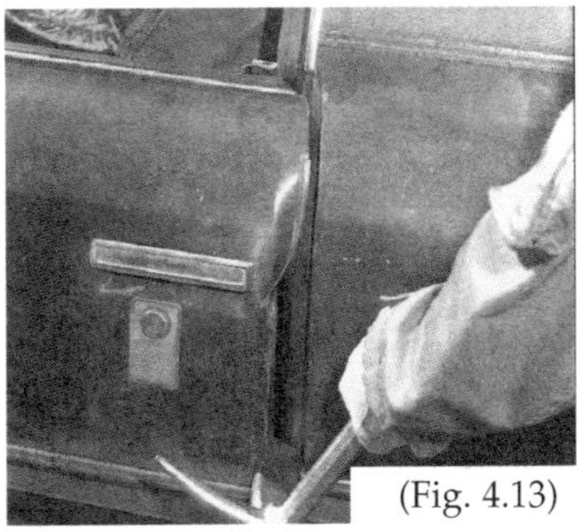

(Fig. 4.13)

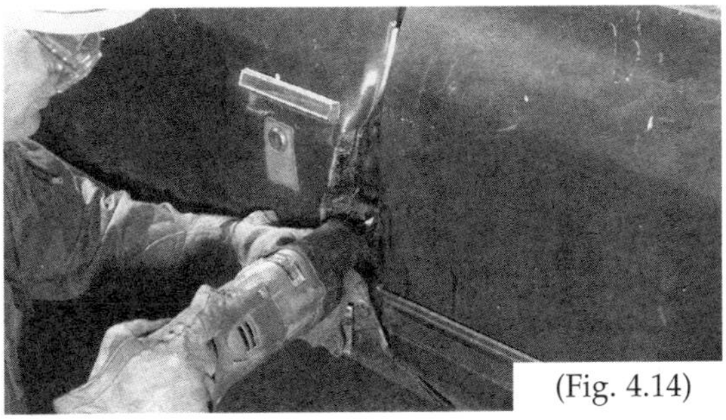

(Fig. 4.14)

Using the reciprocating saw with a small blade, cut through the bolt (Fig. 4.14). Apply the soapy water liberally. The bolt should part in 20 to 30 seconds. Use the halligan tool to force the door past the jam.

You may choose to remove the door from the hinge side. There are two types of hinges: cast and formed or stamped. The cast hinge is the tougher of the two (Fig. 4.15).

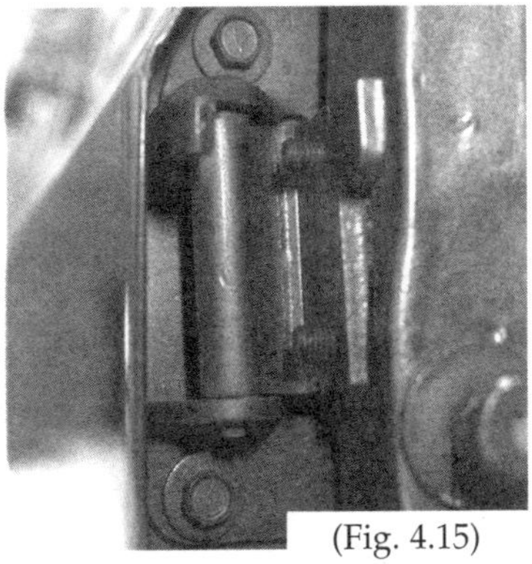

(Fig. 4.15)

The formed or stamped hinge is made of mild steel and is very easy to cut (Fig. 4.16).

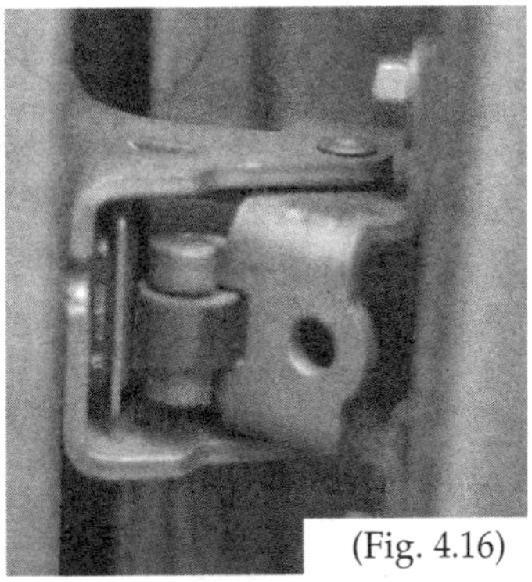

(Fig. 4.16)

The removal techniques are the same. First, you will need to make an opening with the halligan tool to expose the hinges (Fig. 4.17).

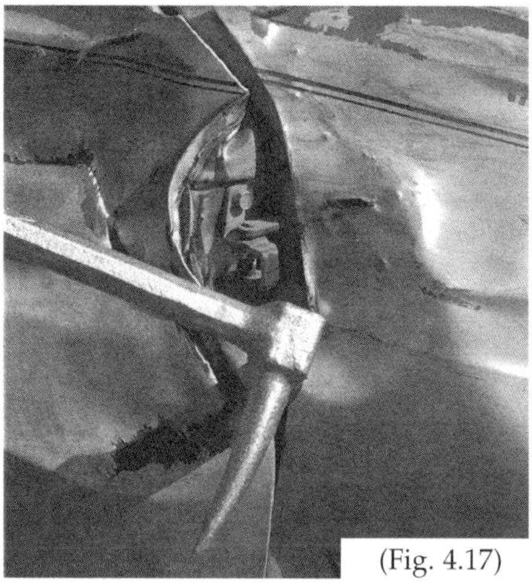

(Fig. 4.17)

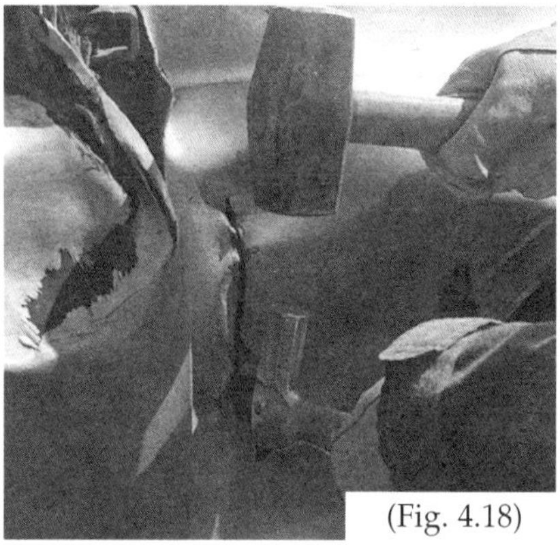

(Fig. 4.18)

Some vehicles may require the use of the panel cutter to accomplish this (Fig. 4.18).

Once exposed, cut the hinges with the reciprocating saw (Fig. 4.19). The size of the blade will be determined after you expose the hinges. In most cases, the short blade is used so as not to "bottom out."

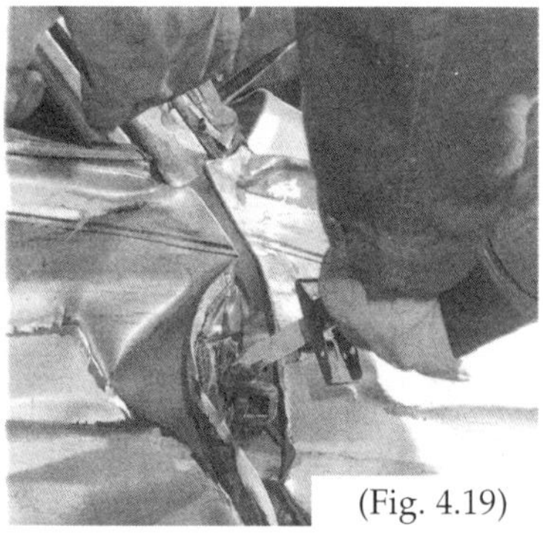

(Fig. 4.19)

Once the hinges are cut, bend the door back on the lock in a circular motion (Fig. 4.20).

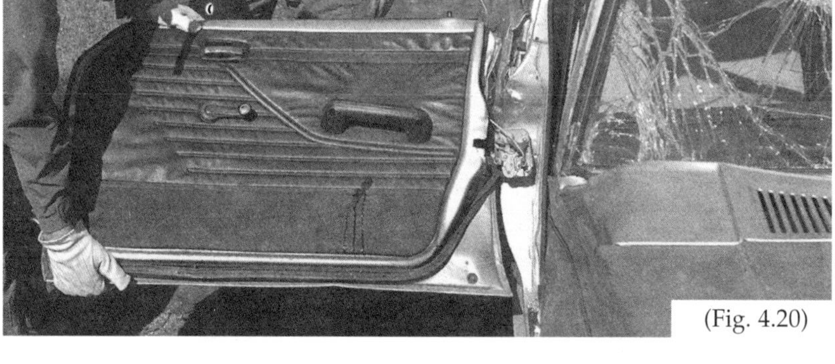

(Fig. 4.20)

In most instances, the bolt will pull loose from the scissors. Be careful! Many times the scissors let go unexpectedly and the door will drop on your feet (Fig. 4.21). Be sure to move the door away from the vehicle so it does not become a tripping hazard.

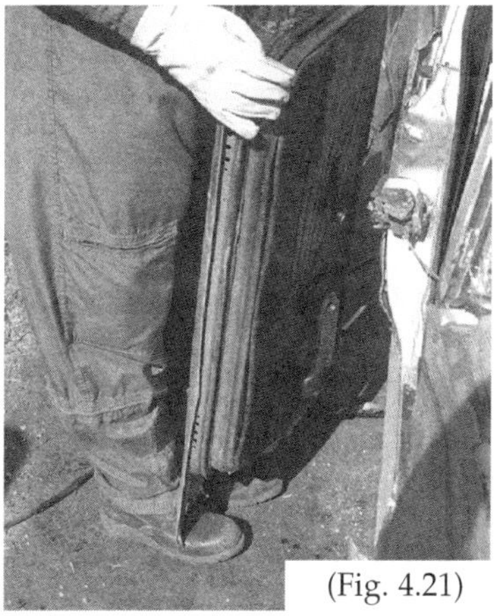

(Fig. 4.21)

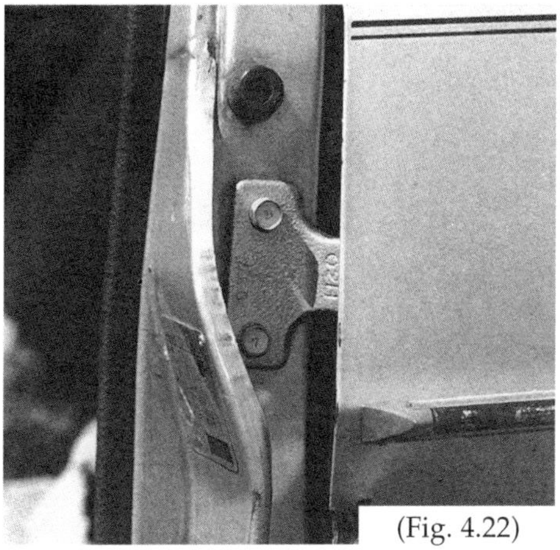

(Fig. 4.22)

Thus far we have only discussed removal of the front doors. The latch/lock is virtually the same on the rear doors. An additional method for removing the rear door is by unbolting it. When the front door is removed on most cars, it reveals the hinges on the rear door (Fig. 4.22).

If you see three bolt heads on each hinge, chances are you can remove them. The bolt size will be 1/2″ or 9/16″ unless it is metric. In which case the size should be 14 or 15 mm.

An open end or box wrench will do the job (Fig. 4.23). Once removed, the hinges will allow the rear door to be twisted on the lock bolt as you did with the front door.

We will discuss removing the entire side or dropping the side under Chapter Six, Disentanglement.

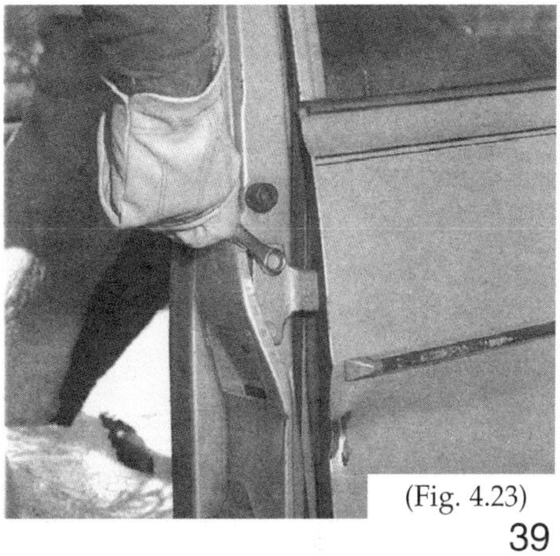

(Fig. 4.23)

ROOFS

For some reason medics try to treat victims in vehicles while the roof remains in place. The vehicle could be a total loss and there's still the hesitation to make room for everyone's safety. Roofs do not grow on cars, they are put on by mechanics at the factory, so too, can mechanics replace a roof in the field at a surprisingly low cost.

There should never be a monetary consideration in deciding when to remove a roof. If the victim is conscious and complains of a neck or back injury, the roof goes! If the victim is unconscious and in a compromised position as to a possible airway, neck or back injury, the roof goes! There isn't any comparison of a Rolls Royce at $ 135,000.00, and a multi-million dollar lawsuit, when a C-spine injury is in question!

The removal procedure is very simple with either a hand-held hacksaw or a reciprocating saw. Much time can be saved if you first open the doors, thus avoiding having to cut the window frames. Start with the "A" pillar and cut at right angles about four inches up from the dash (Fig. 4.24).

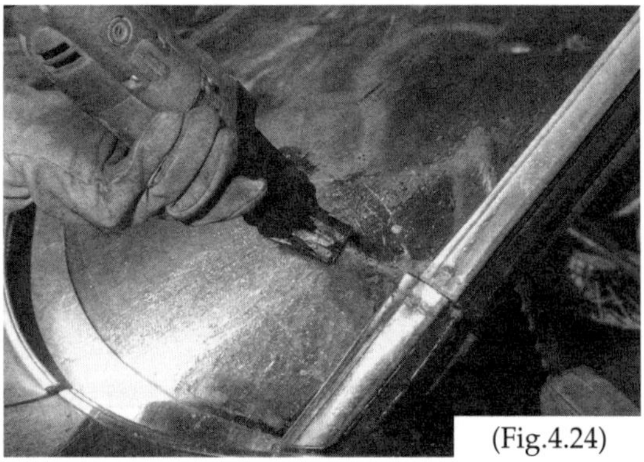

(Fig.4.24)

Cut all the way through to the windshield. Next cut the "B" pillars within two inches of the top. Then the "C" pillars. Here you could have a minor problem if you are using hand hacksaws. Look to see the shortest distance glass to glass (door opening to the rear window).

Start your cut from the front to the rear on an angle (never straight). If the "C" pillar is too wide for the saw frame, cut a pie shaped wedge from the rear and finish off the cut. Take advantage of opera windows in this phase of the cut.

When using the reciprocating saw, work it like a chain saw, up and down, creating a new edge at every stroke. Let the saw do the work while keeping a steady pressure. Your partner should keep a good spray from the soap bottle on the saw blade. The secret to quick cutting is a new blade and solid pressure of the swivel foot to the surface to be cut (Fig. 4.25).

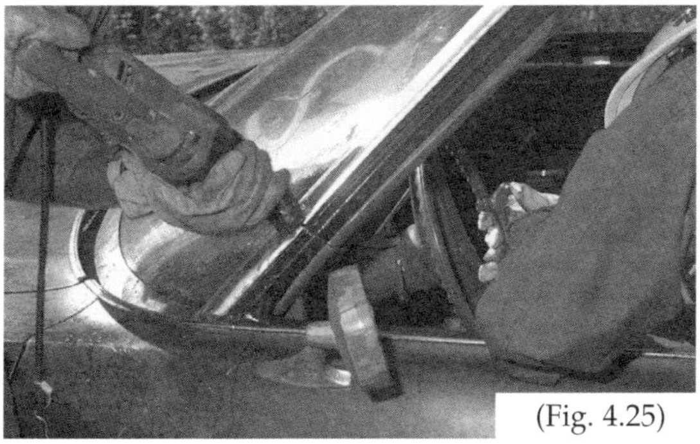

(Fig. 4.25)

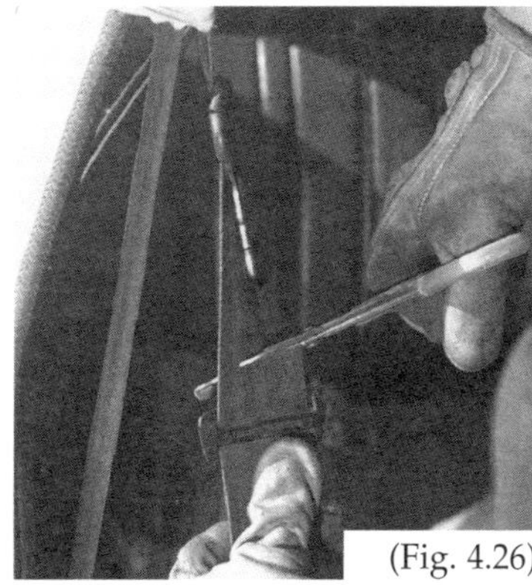

(Fig. 4.26)

When all the pillars are severed, cut the seat belts (Fig. 4.26) and, with your partner on the far side, lift the roof to a vertical position from the rear to the front (Fig. 4.27). The windshield will tear away at the base and the roof will be placed upside down on the hood. By using this method, glass will not pass over the victim(s).

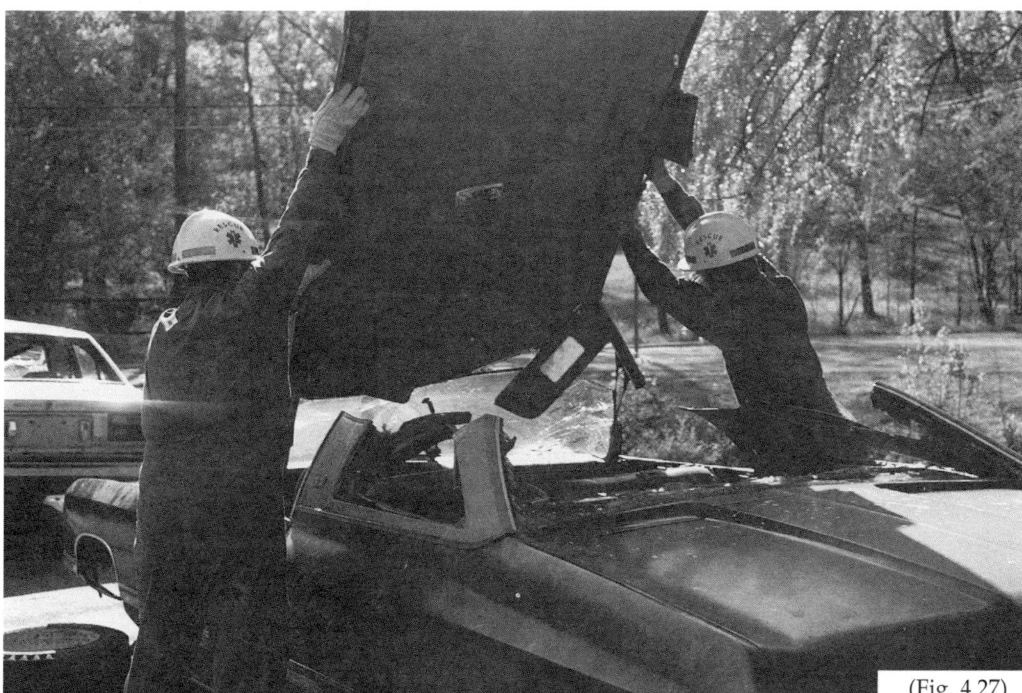

(Fig. 4.27)

It is rather useless to flap a roof, as it takes only a few seconds more to remove it. Be sure to cover any exposed pillar ends with duct tape, so as not to be cut (Fig. 4.28).

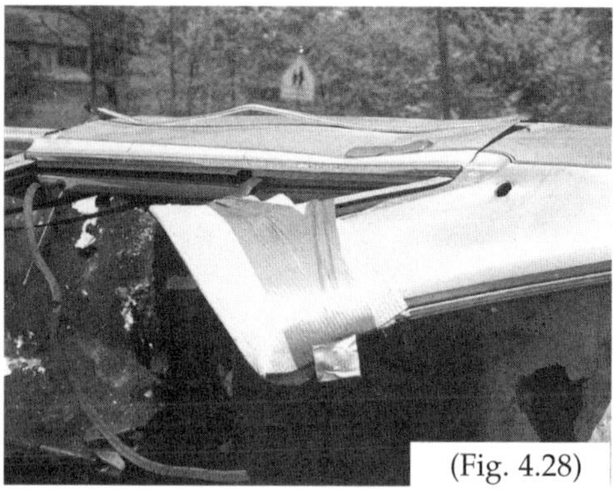

(Fig. 4.28)

The placement of collars and treatment in general is tremendously enhanced when you have room to move around and are able to see what you are doing.

Dropping the Roof of a Car on Its Side

Slide a full spine board into the rear window to protect the victim(s).

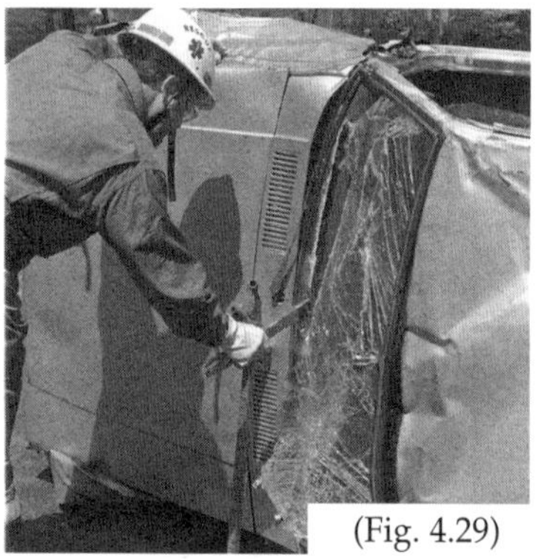

(Fig. 4.29)

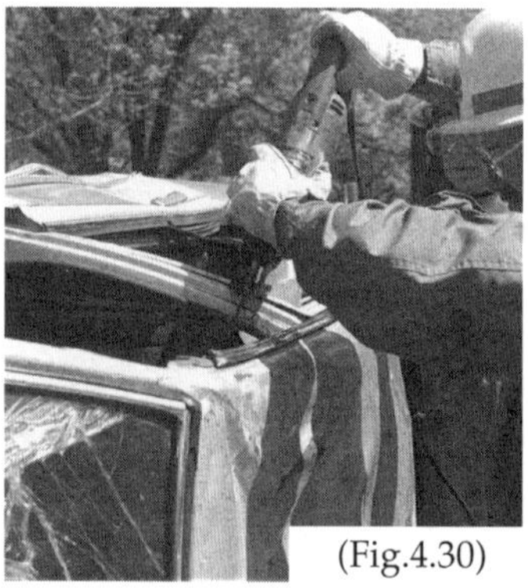

(Fig.4.30)

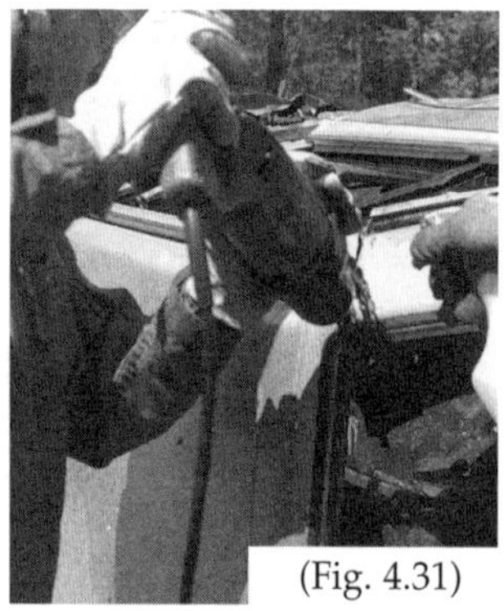

(Fig. 4.31)

Cut the uppermost "A" (Fig. 4.29), "B" (if there is one) (Fig. 4.30), and "C" pillars (Fig. 4.31) as you did on the car on its wheels.

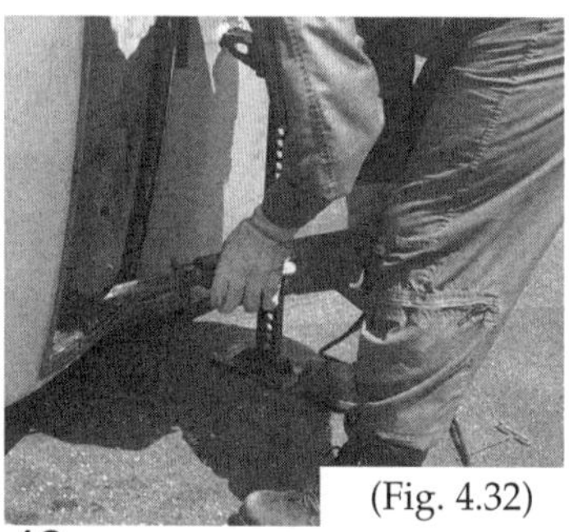

(Fig. 4.32)

When cutting the "A" pillar, allow the saw to cut the bottom of the windshield all the way to the lower "A" pillar. Cut this pillar half way through (Fig. 4.32). Remove any tempered glass that may be in your way in both the side or rear windows.

Reach in and cut the "B" pillar (if there is one) half way through and repeat on the "C" pillar (Fig. 4.33).

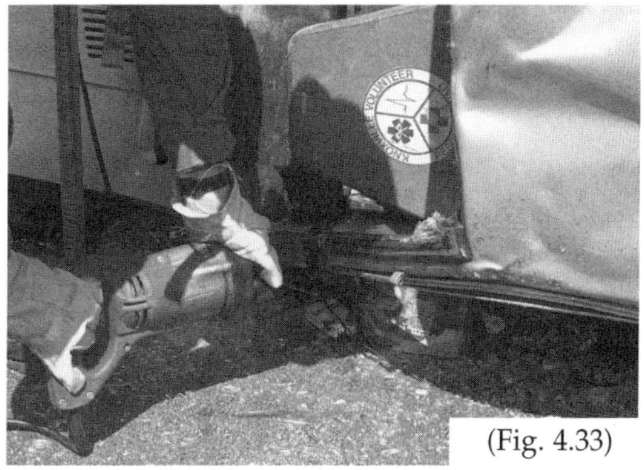

(Fig. 4.33)

All these "halfway" cuts are from the inside down toward the outside, so you can bend the entire roof downward (Fig. 4.34), (after having cut the upper seat belt).

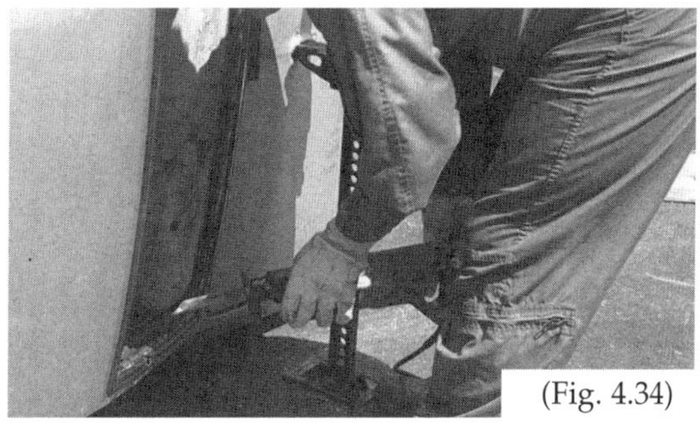

(Fig. 4.34)

This will insure the stability of the car as the roof will not be entirely removed (Fig. 4.35).

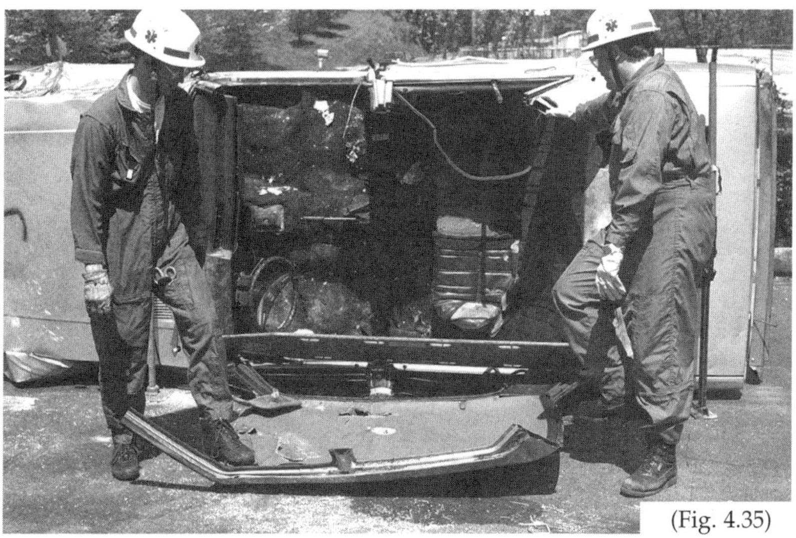

(Fig. 4.35)

Cover all sharp edges of the severed pillars with duct tape, hose sections, multi-trauma dressings, etc. (Fig. 4.36).

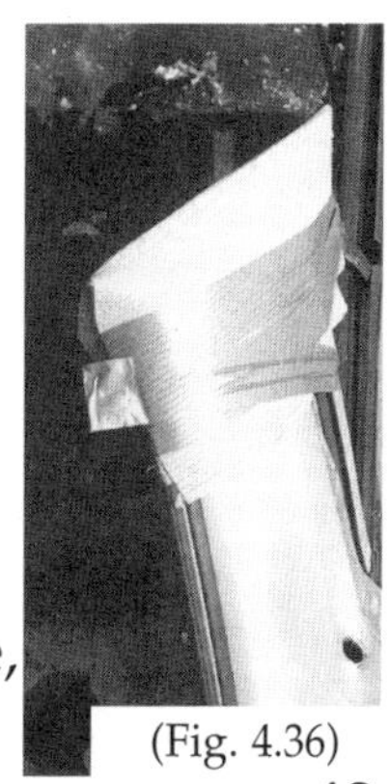

(Fig. 4.36)

FLOORS

Probably the softest part of the car is the floor assembly. The vehicle may come to rest on it's side into a building, upside down in a ditch, or in some other position in which you are confronted with accessing through the bottom of the vehicle, as the doors or roof are inaccessible.

The first step is to clean off the bottom of the vehicle. Using the power saw, cut the drive shaft at the universal joint and pull it toward the rear to slide it out of the spline in the transmission and discard it. Next, cut the brake cables and cut off the exhaust system. Be careful that the catalytic converter does not burn you.

The foot well in the rear seat is very obvious when viewed from the bottom. Punch out the drain hole covers to give yourself an opening for the reciprocating saw (Fig. 4.37).

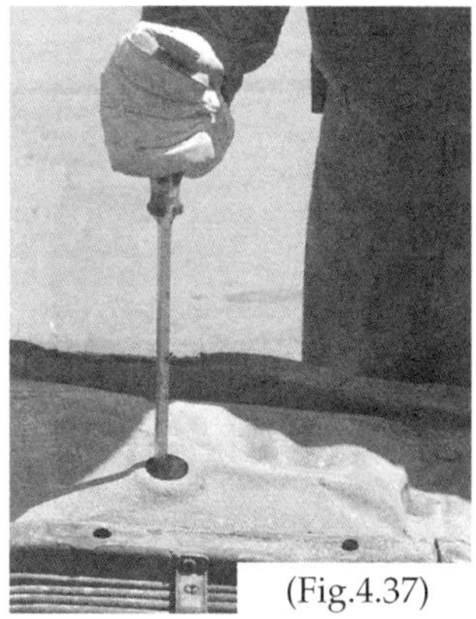

(Fig.4.37)

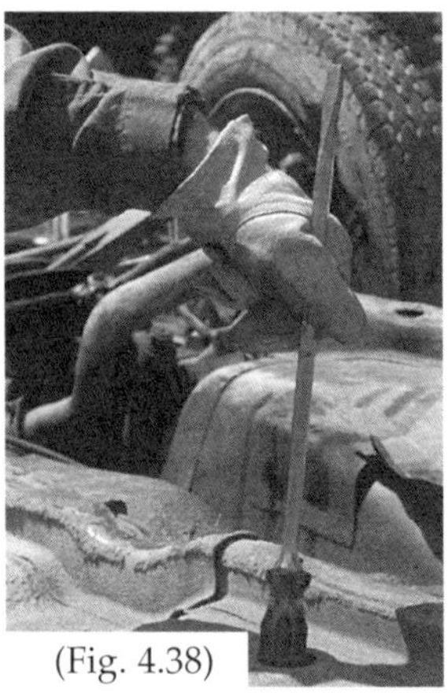

(Fig. 4.38)

Be sure to use the short saw blade. Push the handle of the large screwdriver through the hole to make sure no body parts are near the intended saw path (Fig. 4.38).

Remember, you are under the rug so there should not be a problem. Make a three-sided cut the full size of the raised portion of the floor pan (Fig. 4.39).

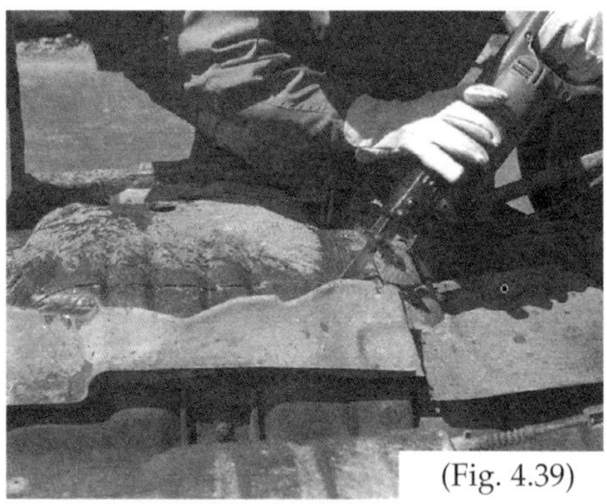

(Fig. 4.39)

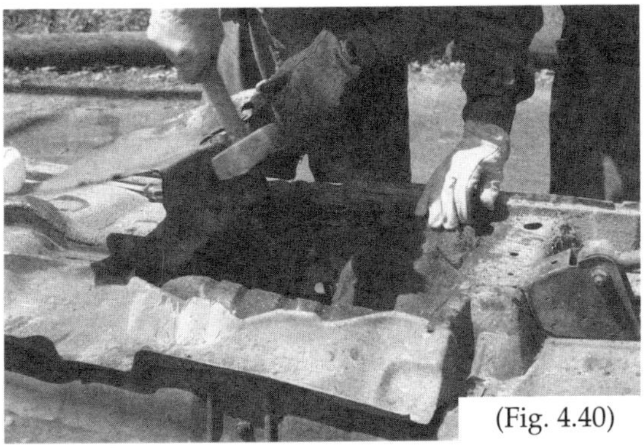

(Fig. 4.40)

Bend back the flap and push the rug in and out of the way (Fig. 4.40). At this time, you should be able to determine if any of the victims are in the way.

You or your partner can crawl through the opening to stabilize the victim(s),(Fig.4.41). Make sure you run duct tape around the sharp edges of the opening before entering.

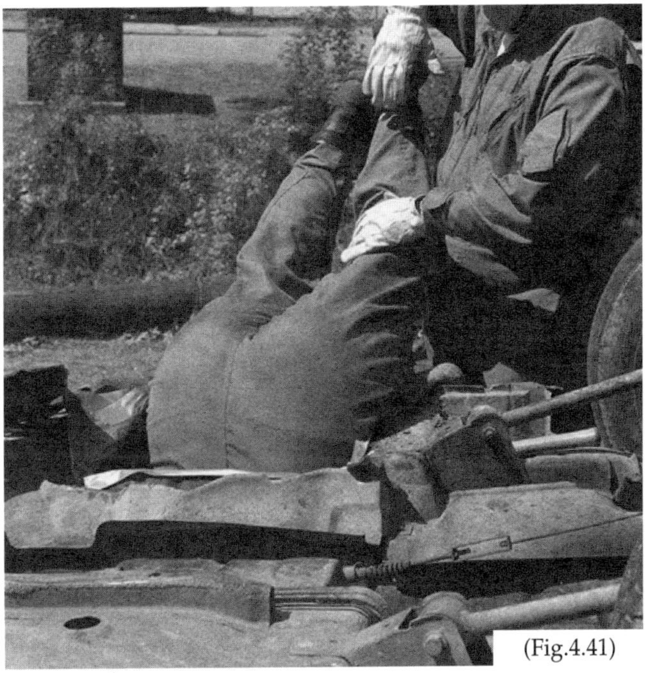

(Fig.4.41)

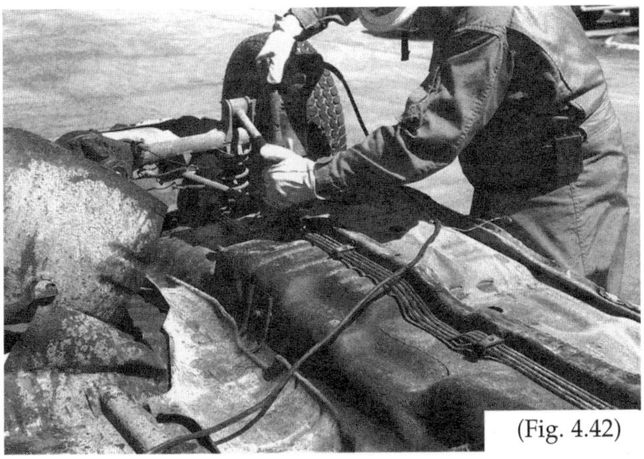

(Fig. 4.42)

When removing the entire floor, the reciprocating saw is run around the perimeter of the passenger compartment (Fig. 4.42). The only problems normally encountered are around the transmission; it may be necessary to cut the support brackets

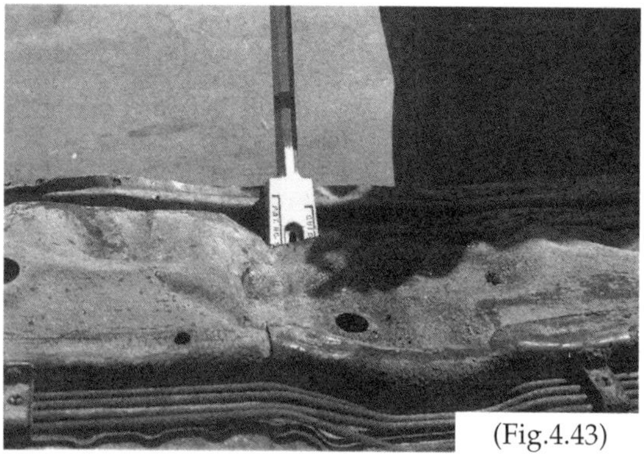
(Fig.4.43)

Next, cut the seat belts to the front seat and with the long pinch bar and halligan tool (Fig. 4.43)

Pry the entire floor out from the car along with the front seat attached. You will then have the entire passenger compartment exposed.

ENGINE COMPARTMENT

Be aware the firewalls on most vehicles have large holes in them to accommodate heater/air conditioning components, and these are usually made of plastic (Fig. 4.44).

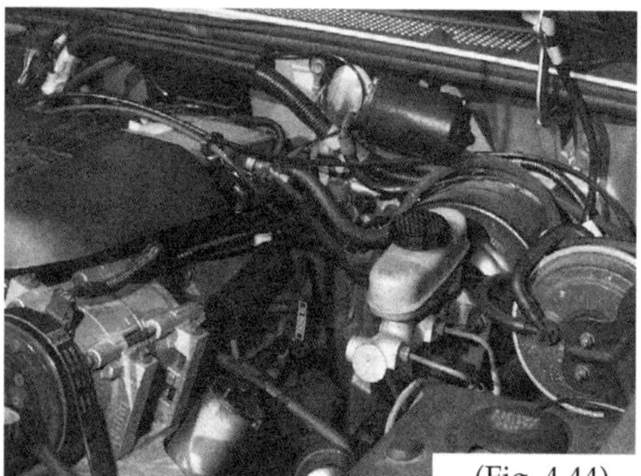
(Fig. 4.44)

The transfer of heat, smoke and fire can occur very rapidly from the engine compartment into the passenger area. It is therefore imperative that a fire be stopped in its incipient stage when persons are trapped.

Immediately upon arrival, try to pop the hood of the vehicle if smoke is showing around it. Have your partner stand by with an ABC extinguisher. If the fire is of any severity, the hood latch mechanism has long since melted off.

Do not waste time trying to force the hood. Using the pike end of the halligan tool, drive it through the hood in at least four places, one foot on either side of the center (Fig. 4.45). This will assure that you miss the air cleaner.

Next, push the long screwdriver through the holes to free them of insulation.

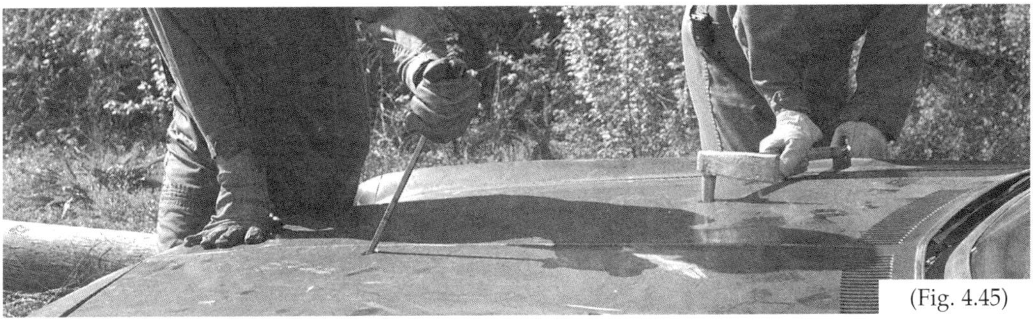

(Fig. 4.45)

Hold the extinguisher nozzle in the holes and discharge it in short bursts (Fig. 4.46).

If a garden hose is available nearby, use it!

The threat of fire is the one time that all other actions are put aside to concentrate on the victim(s) removal. While one medic tries to contain the fire, the other works on the victim(s).

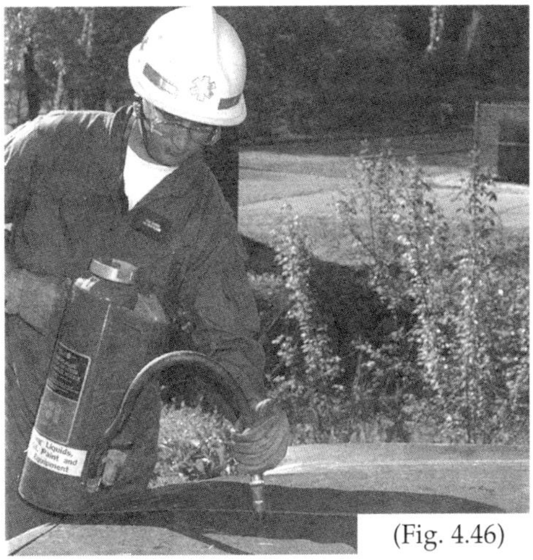

(Fig. 4.46)

TRUNK COMPARTMENT

The trunk can be quite hazardous in that people tend to use it as a storage locker.

Flammable materials such as books, papers, cartons, clothing, gasoline and explosive materials such as spare tires, air cans, aerosol cans and many others too numerous to mention can create a hazmat condition. Here again, the transfer of a fire into the passenger compartment would be quicker than the front end, as it is usually wide open behind the rear seat cushion.

In case there is a fire, do not open the trunk, as this would be just the time one of these "hazmats" would explode causing serious injury. Instead, using the pinch bar or halligan tool, smash out the rear lights — they usually extend into the trunk compartment. Next, spray an extinguishing agent through the opening (Fig. 4.47).

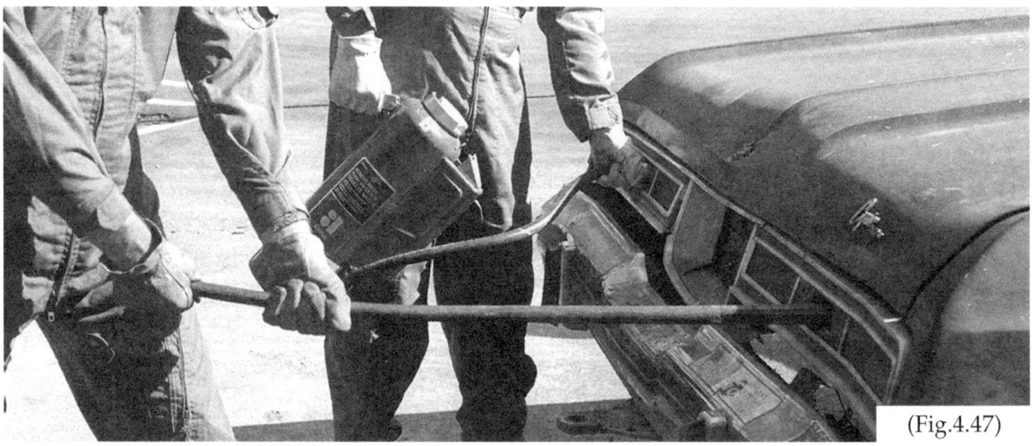

(Fig.4.47)

Once again, while one medic is taking care of this task, the other is working to free and remove the victim(s).

One more thing concerning the trunk. Never leave the scene of any accident without first checking all vehicle trunks of the cars involved. It is entirely possible that persons could be in the trunk at the time of the accident and be knocked unconscious. College hazing is just one example of why the victim could be locked in the trunk.

KEY POINTS TO REMEMBER

- Note the placement of the center punch at the lower corner of the window. This restricts "follow through" of the hand.
- When using a striking tool to break glass, the motion should be with the wrist.
- All glass will cut when broken.
- Doors are the preferred mode of entry and egress.
- If doors are jammed on one side, try the other side before starting forcible entry.
- No amount of force on a pry bar will break the door latch!
- When cutting anything, lubricate liberally with soapy water.
- Use a generic dishwashing detergent mixed with water, 6 to 1, put the water in the spray bottle first and add the detergent to prevent suds.
- Use a small (4") saw blade if the problem of "bottoming out" is a possibility.
- Cast hinges are harder to cut than stamped or pressed hinges. Be careful that door does not drop if a cast hinge shatters.
- Roof removal gives much more room to provide patient care, protect the C-spine and secure the airway.
- Flapping the roof requires more effort and time than removing it altogether.

- **It is usually not necessary to cut the bottom of the windshield when removing the roof from rear to front. The windshield will tear away. This will also reduce the risk of glass falling on your patient.**

- **All gas lines must be cut and plugged before stripping the vehicle bottom.**

- **If gas lines are metal, crimp them with pliers before cutting.**

- **Be aware that catalytic converters can be extremely hot.**

NOTES:

JOTTING DOWN IMPORTANT INFORMATION WILL HELP YOU REMEMBER AND EXPAND YOUR KNOWLEDGE

SPACE FOR NOTES IS PROVIDED AFTER EACH CHAPTER FOR YOU TO ADD YOUR OWN "BITS AND PIECES" OF INFORMATION.

CHAPTER FIVE

STABILIZING THE VICTIM

KNOWLEDGE OBJECTIVES:
The rescuer should be able to...

- **Summarize activities of the stabilization of victims;**
- **Describe the steps of the in-vehicle emergency care procedures;**
- **Describe steps that can be used to protect the victim from further injury.**

SKILL OBJECTIVES:
The rescuer should be able to...

- **Carry out the in vehicle emergency care procedures;**
- **Protect the victim from further injury.**

CHAPTER FIVE

STABILIZING THE VICTIM

OK, you have gained access. At this point, I will make a few comments and then back-off to allow you to practice your medical expertise. Your job now is to keep the victim(s) alive, while you think ahead as to how you will extricate and package the person(s) in anticipation of removal.

Certainly we all know enough to maintain an open airway and control bleeding, while applying a cervical collar. Kid stuff! Right? Wrong! Too many times EMS units are not taught under realistic conditions. We have gotten away from showing "blood and guts" type films and slides in training exercises. Thus, the first few times answering a particularly bloody call, many crews become traumatized themselves. How many have been taught how to apply a cervical collar while sitting upright in a kitchen chair? This is totally unrealistic. Try practicing on real people in various pretzel-like positions in wrecked cars. Quite a difference!

Your assessment of the victim(s) should follow the steps outlined in the BTLS primary and secondary survey. The BTLS primary survey is designed to identify those problems that pose an immediate threat to the victim's life.

Assess the airway for patency. If it is not patent, open the airway using the chin-lift, jaw-thrust method. Any obstructions, such as blood, vomitus or foreign bodies, must be cleared, using suction or the obstructed airway maneuver. All trauma victims should receive supplemental oxygen.

Breathing is assessed for rate and adequacy. If the breathing is inadequate, assist the victim's respiration with a bag-valve mask (BVM). If the victim is unable to protect their airway (absent gag) or there is a significant risk of losing the airway, you must secure the airway using endotracheal intubation, a blind insertion airway device (BIAD) or other airway adjunct, dependent upon what your level of training permits you to do.

Listen to the chest for presence of breath sounds. Absent breath sounds and tracheal deviation away from the injured side are signs of a tension pneumothorax. This should be relieved by needle decompression, as soon as possible.

Assess the circulation by checking for presence of both a carotid and radial pulse. Absence of a radial pulse, with carotid pulses present indicates that the victim may be going into shock. Also remember that a rapid pulse in the presence of good perfusion may represent the earliest sign of shock. IV access and fluid resuscitation should not be attempted in the vehicle, unless you are faced with a prolonged extrication problem. In critical victims, IV's should be started enroute to the hospital.

Assess the neurologic status of the victim to stimuli, using the AVPU method. Altered level of consciousness may be due to head trauma, poor perfusion or hypoxia. Do not assume that the victim is unconscious "because they are drunk."

The primary survey should take less than ninety (90) seconds, in most cases. It should be interrupted only to correct potentially life threatening conditions that have been identified in the primary survey. Remember that any victim with a problem identified in the primary survey should be classified as a "Load and Go," requiring rapid extrication and prompt transport.

This is only a brief overview of assessment and stabilization. For a more complete explanation of the process, you should review your BTLS Textbook. Remember also, that while assessment and stabilization have begun during this phase of the rescue, they must be continued throughout the rest of the rescue and during transport to the hospital.

Protecting the Victim

Many times no thought is given to the victim as far as protecting them from further injury. Now that you are inside the vehicle and doing a primary survey on the victim, you will have to determine what extra measures you must take to protect the head, eyes, ears, etc. Make sure the victim(s) are shielded from glass fragments. Use a blanket, tarpaulin, turn-out coat or even a newspaper found in the vehicle.

KEY POINTS TO REMEMBER

- Primary Survey:
  - "A" - Airway with C-spine protection
  - "B" - Breathing assessment and support
  - "C" - Circulatory assessment and support

Any problem identified in the primary survey means that the patient meets "Load and Go" criteria!

- Do not delay transport except to secure airway. IV's should be established enroute to the hospital, unless there is going to be a prolonged extrication.

- Absence of a radial pulse suggest shock.

- Mental status exam:
  - "A" - Victim is ALERT
  - "V" - Victim responds to VERBAL stimuli
  - "P" - Victim responds to PAIN
  - "U" - Victim is UNRESPONSIVE

  - Drunks do die!

  - Care of the victim is an on-going process.

  - Reassess victim frequently.

  - Provide psychological support:

    Talk to the victim.
    Tell him what is happening.

  - Watch for Hypothermia in victims and personnel.

NOTES:

JOTTING DOWN IMPORTANT INFORMATION WILL HELP YOU REMEMBER AND EXPAND YOUR KNOWLEDGE

SPACE FOR NOTES IS PROVIDED AFTER EACH CHAPTER FOR YOU TO ADD YOUR OWN "BITS AND PIECES" OF INFORMATION.

CHAPTER SIX

DISENTANGLEMENT

KNOWLEDGE OBJECTIVES:

The rescuer should be able to...

- Summarize the disentanglement phase of vehicle rescue;
- Describe removing the battery cable;
- Describe methods of removal from steering column/wheel entrapment;
- Describe "blowing out" the front end of the vehicle;
- Describe disentangling a trapped foot;
- Describe dropping the sides of a wrecked vehicle;
- Describe lifting a vehicle off a trapped victim.

SKILL OBJECTIVES:

The rescuer should be able to...

- Remove the correct battery cable;
- Correctly move back a seat;
- Remove the steering wheel rim;
- Remove the steering column;
- "Blow out" the front end;
- Disentangle a trapped foot;
- Drop the sides of a wrecked vehicle;
- Lift a vehicle off a victim underneath.

CHAPTER SIX

DISENTANGLEMENT

In the case of BTLS Access, disentangling is literally freeing the victim from the wreckage. We can liken it to peeling an orange. It is very seldom that the victim is impaled, rather, the entrapment results from the wreckage being wrapped around the victim.

Disentanglement then is the prelude to packaging. The moving of metal or plastic to allow the easy movement of the victim.

We have already discussed the removal of the roof and doors to gain access, now, let's discuss techniques which will quicken the "freeing" process.

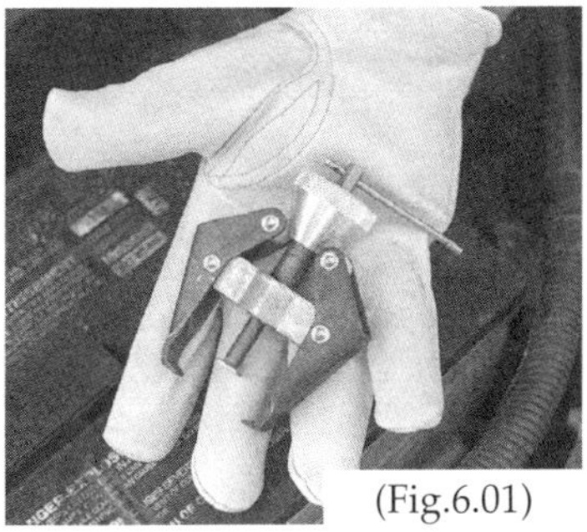

(Fig.6.01)

You will note in your tool kit, a battery cable puller (Fig. 6.01).

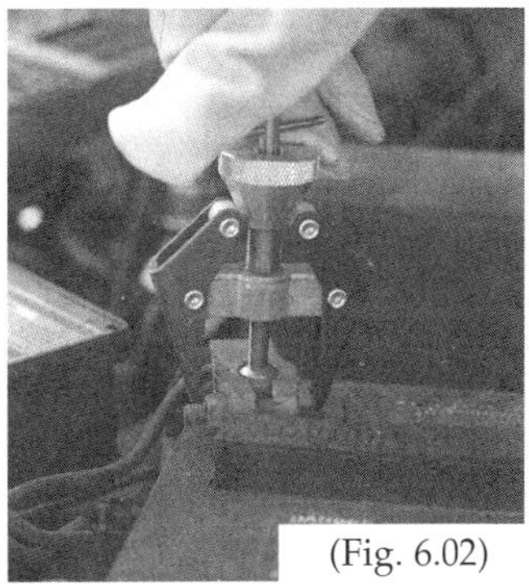

(Fig. 6.02)

Do not cut the battery cables. Remove the negative cable (black) if you are experiencing an electrical problem (Fig. 6.02), or to cancel the airbags if they were not deployed. If you have no apparent problems, do not touch the battery! Today's automobiles have too many functions which rely on electric power, to have an SOP which calls for disconnecting power indiscriminately.

If you cannot obtain a battery puller, use battery pliers (Fig. 6.03).

You will know when to remove the cable(s) without me telling you, common sense prevails in this case!

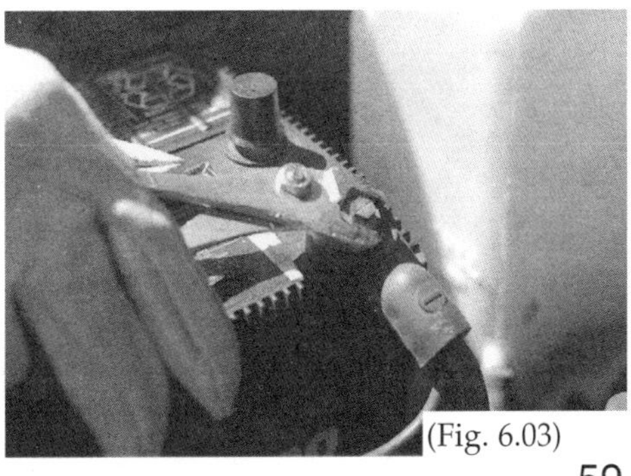

(Fig. 6.03)

Steering Column / Wheel

Probably the most common cause of entrapment is the steering column/wheel. The old "rig from the frame and pull it out like a bad tooth with a tool on the hood" routine is just that, OLD. Though never say never, there are many more sophisticated ways to solve the problem.

First, have you tried the seat? If it is a mechanical bench seat, it may have slipped the ratchet and moved forward during the crash. Have your partner grasp the seat with both hands (one on front of the seat and one on the top of the back). Trip the seat adjustment lever (remember, the seat is sprung to move forward) (Fig. 6.04), and gently push the seat back.

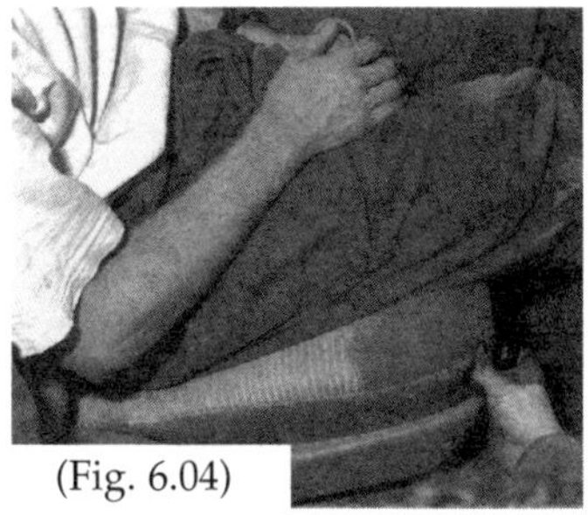

(Fig. 6.04)

A jerky motion which can be accentuated by the spring action could seriously jeopardize a C-spine injury. If the seat is a mechanical bucket seat, the same rules apply.

Do not attempt to move the seat back by yourself.

If the seat is electrically operated, find the right button to move it back (Fig. 6.05).

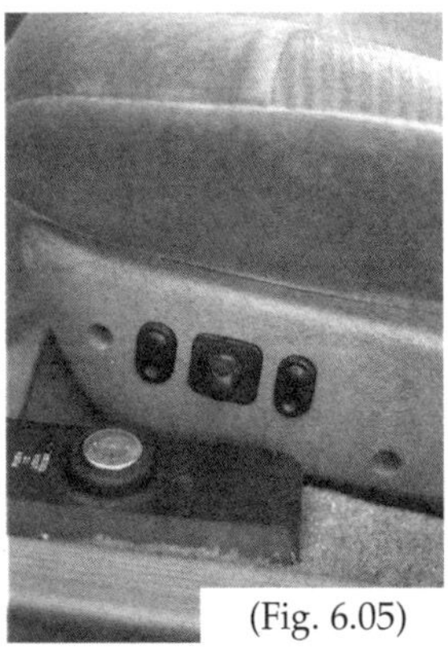

(Fig. 6.05)

Read the directional labels so as not to aggravate the situation by pushing the wrong button. Never attempt to dislodge the seat with mechanical force (hydraulic tools) with the victim on it.

Six to eight inches can be gained by moving a seat back. If you are not successful, the next step is to remove the steering wheel.

The rim of a steering wheel can be cut easily with either the hand or power saws (Fig. 6.06). The metal used on the rim is soft steel with no spring action.

Either cut the spokes or bend them out of the way. This action will gain an additional six inches (Fig. 6.07).

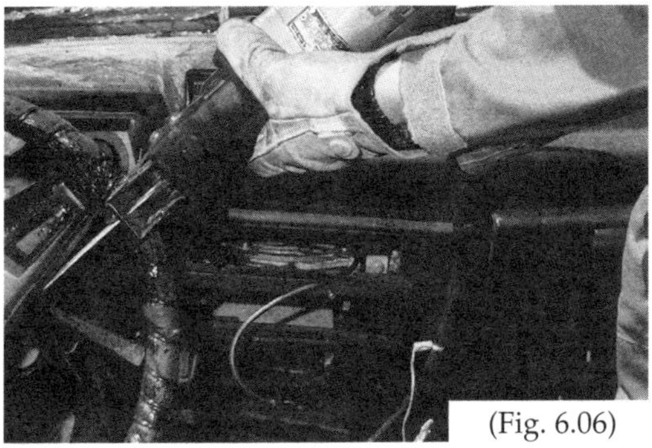

(Fig. 6.06)

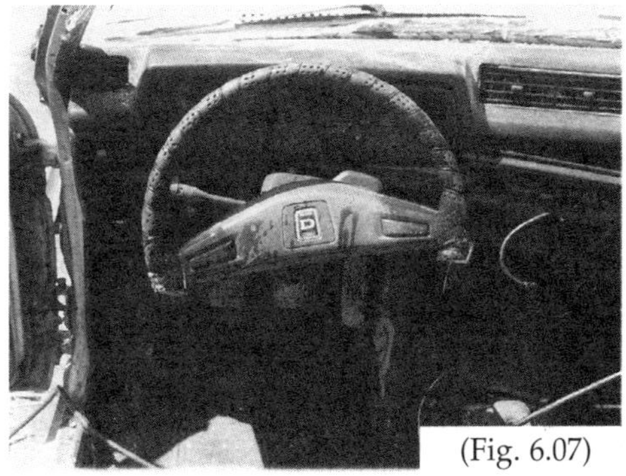

(Fig. 6.07)

If the car is equipped with an undeployed air bag, disconnect the battery terminals and work around the bag module. Do not cut into the module, it will serve no purpose.

Still not enough room? We can remove the steering column, not by pulling, but by cutting! Though the columns on some cars look awesome because of their size, you must realize the actual steering column is nothing more than a 5/8″ or 3/4″ mild steel shaft easily cut with the hand saw or power saw once it is stripped.

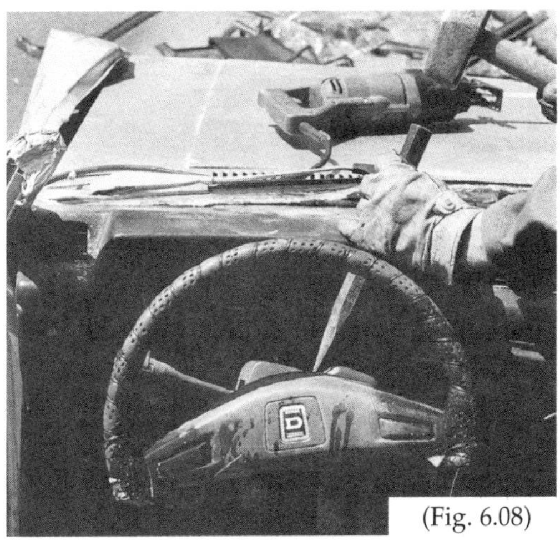

(Fig. 6.08)

Use the cold chisel and machinist hammer to peel off the cosmetic plastics (Fig. 6.08).

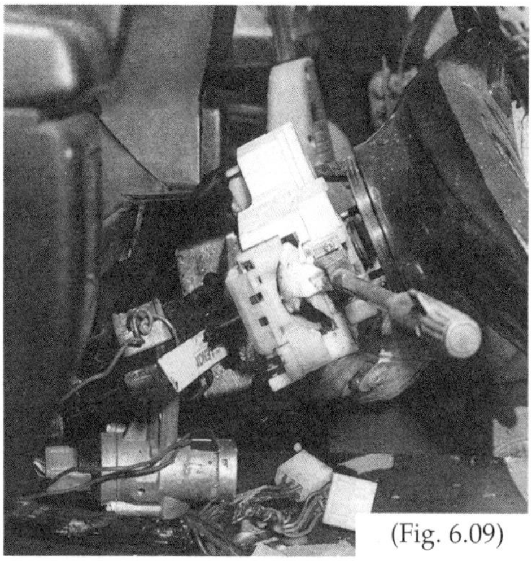

(Fig. 6.09)

You may note the wiring harness runs down the column. (Fig.6.09)

Again, a reason to disconnect the battery cable to avoid any sparking when you cut through the harness. This also prevents the remote possibility of hot-starting the car.

Two things to consider. Be sure the victim is protected before you start cutting. A short back board across the legs will suffice. As an added safety, pull the saw up toward you (this may not be possible, thus the board). Have your partner hold the wheel/column so it does not drop when the cut is through (Fig. 6.10).

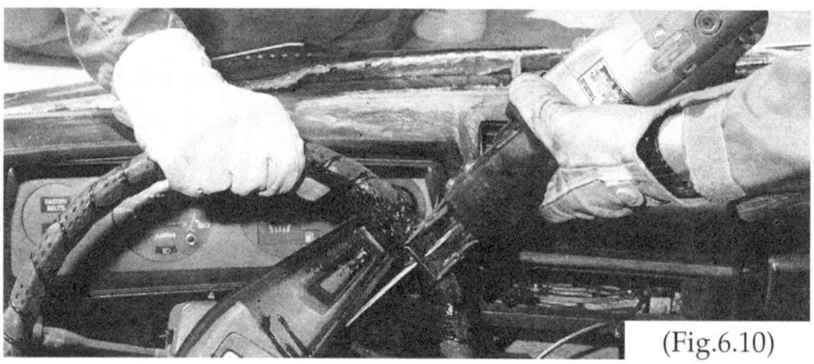

(Fig.6.10)

Be sure to use liberal amounts of soapy water on the saw blade.

Moving the Dash / Front End

There may come a time when the dash is crushed over, preventing all of the above. The answer here is to "blow" the front end out of the car. To even consider a "dash roll" is a waste of time, as was pointed out, flapping the roof versus removal.

Blowing the front end is a very simple maneuver. The roof has been removed and the doors are open or removed as well.

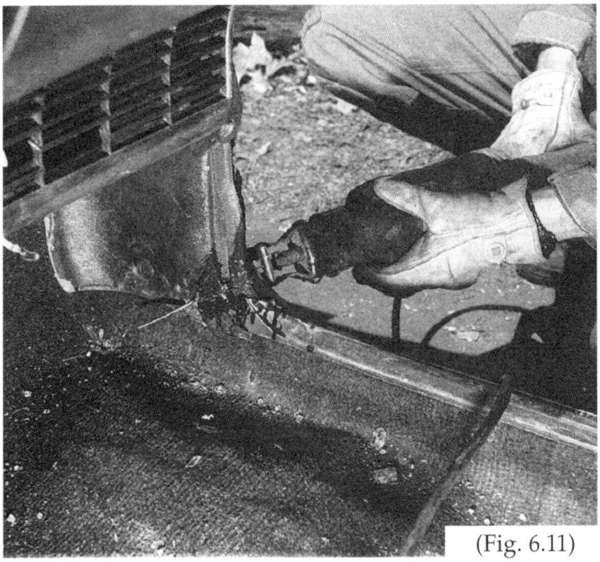

(Fig. 6.11)

Next, using the power saw with the long blade, cut on an angle at the base of the "A" pillars toward the front of the vehicle (Fig. 6.11).

Cut as deep as you can. On a framed auto, only cut the body work, do not attempt to cut the frame.

Place the Hi-Lift Jack with its base against the bottom of the "B" pillar and the lifting lip near the top hinge on the "A" pillar (Fig. 6.12).

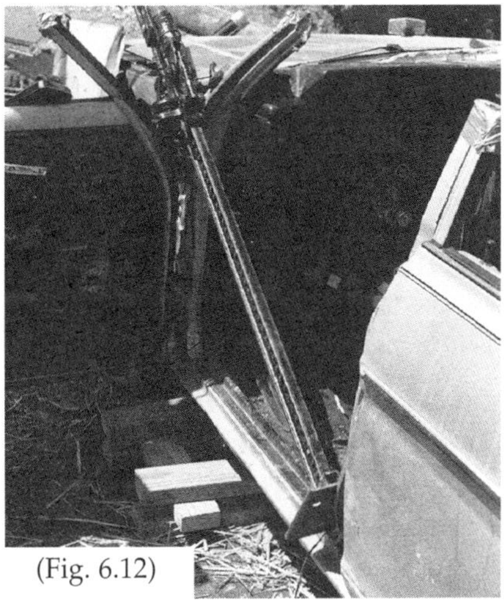

(Fig. 6.12)

If available, a bumper jack can be placed in a similar position on the opposite side.

Use the Hi-Lift on the side the victim is located so as to get maximum push. (Fig. 6.13)

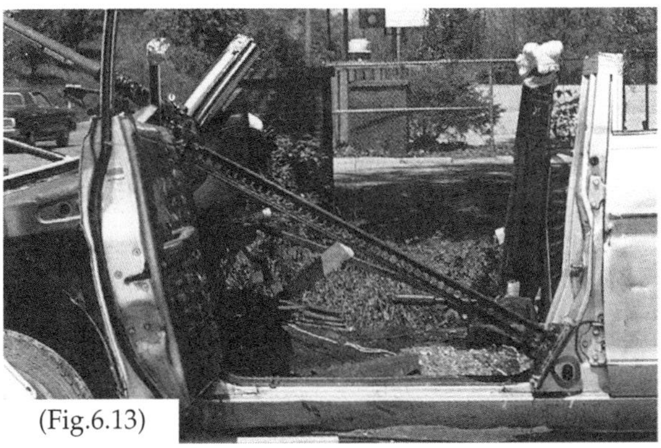

(Fig.6.13)

Work both jacks simultaneously.

The metal at the bottom cuts should start tearing almost immediately.

You must keep checking the lower extremities of the victim to make sure they do not hang up on the column or pedals.

As you jack, crib under the "A" pillars (Fig. 6.14). Only go as far as you need to free the victim.

Remember, a cardinal rule of rescue: "If you need an inch, you do not go two inches, or you are subjecting the victim and yourself to injury!!"

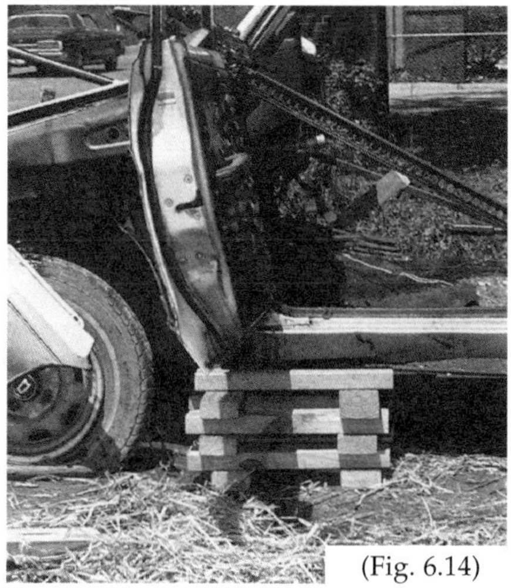

(Fig. 6.14)

Foot / Floorboard Entrapment

Seeming to become more common is the encasing of the foot when the metal floor section folds up under the dash. If the shoe cannot be loosened and the foot slipped out, use the reciprocating saw to cut around the foot and remove the floorboard and victim. Keep well away from the foot when cutting. This may be a time to use the soapy water as a means to slide the foot free. If an opening to start the saw cannot be found, use the Schild panel cutter and machinist hammer to start a slot for the saw blade.

Dropping the Sides

After the roof has been removed, it may be decided to drop the entire side or sides of the vehicle.

By notching the bottom of the "B" pillar front and back (Fig. 6.15) and then slipping the long pinch bar into the top of the pillar (Fig. 6.16) with the round side down, enough leverage can be applied to take the side to the ground (Fig. 6.17).

This can be accomplished with the doors still attached by simply cutting the hinges on the front door and unlatching the rear door. This is the reason we have cut the "B" pillars high when removing the roof. It gives us a great strength and leverage advantage with a longer "B" post.

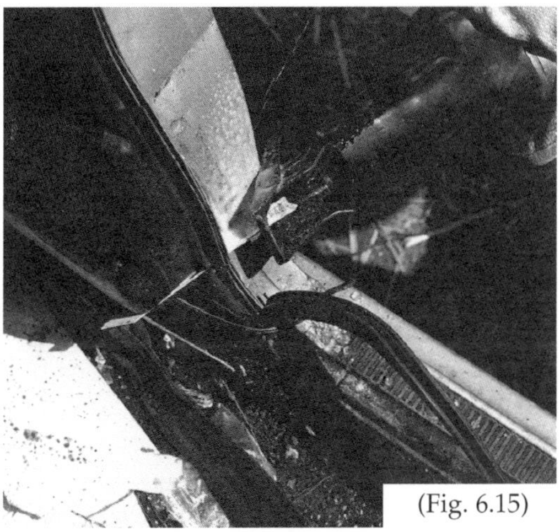
(Fig. 6.15)

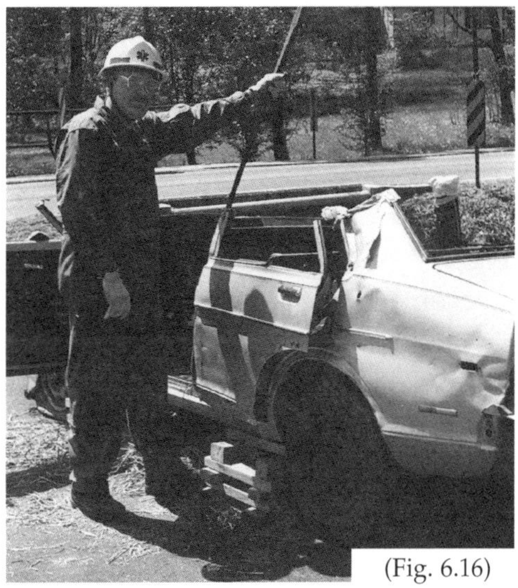
(Fig. 6.16)

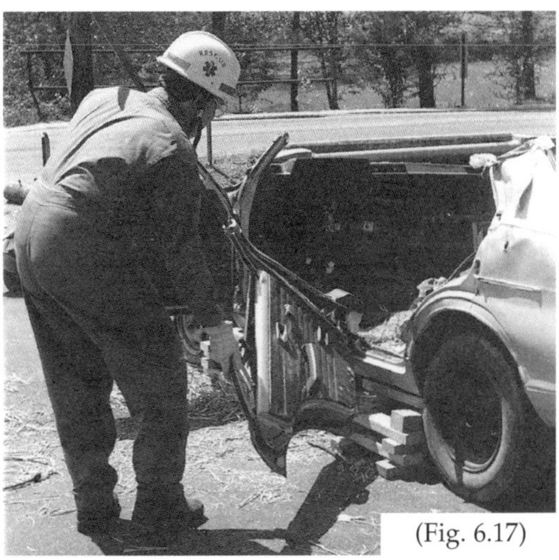
(Fig. 6.17)

Work the pinch bar down into the pillar and pull very easy until you break the back of the "B" pillar. It will tear apart where you notched it.

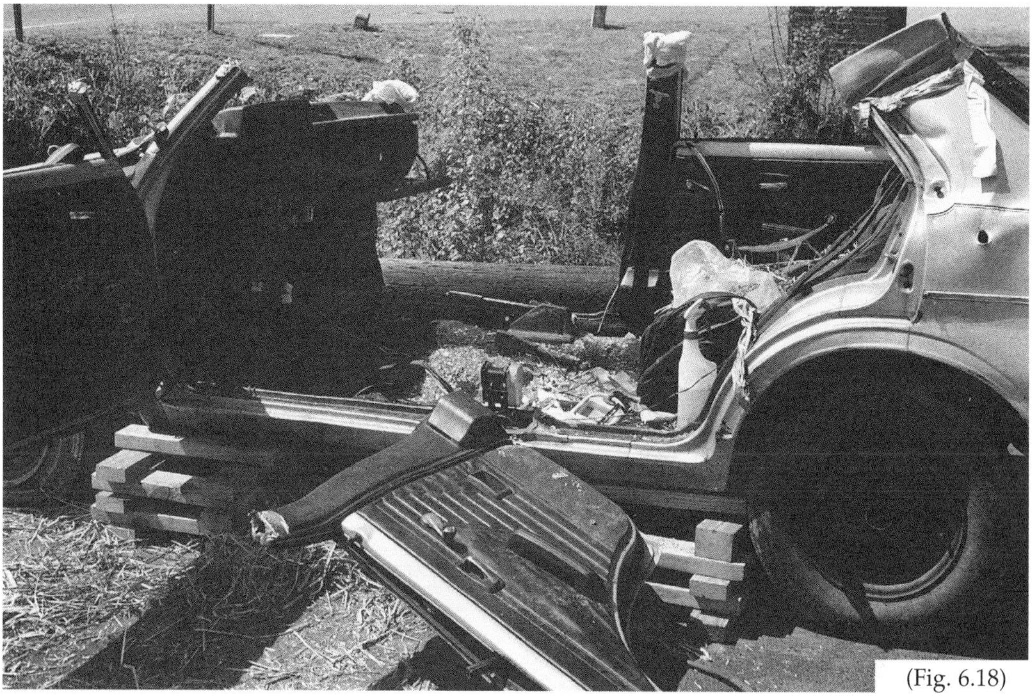

(Fig. 6.18)

The entire interior of the vehicle has now been exposed (Fig. 6.18). The ease of treatment and packaging has been increased one hundred fold. Go get 'em!

Car on Its Wheels — Victim Underneath

In the case of a "backyard mechanic," who has the car fall on him, a different approach must be made.

Chock the car as before. Build box cribs on the side away from the victim's head (opposite the side you will remove the victim from). Lift the side slightly to slide cribbing under the car. Move to the other side of the vehicle and with the Hi-Lift Jack under one wheel well and a bumper jack under the other (same side), jack the vehicle in unison very slowly, cribbing up tight as you go until the victim is free.

Check the far side to make sure you are not sliding off the cribbing. Never flatten the tires when a victim is under the vehicle.

KEY POINTS TO REMEMBER

- **Protect victims at all times when cutting.**

- **Do not pull the steering column:**

  It is dangerous.
  It is unnecessary.
  It takes too long.

- **Always be aware that tools and jacks can slip. Place them carefully.**

- **If you need an inch, do not go two inches!**

- **Cutting the "B" pillars high gives you more leverage when dropping the side.**

NOTES:

JOTTING DOWN IMPORTANT INFORMATION WILL HELP YOU REMEMBER AND EXPAND YOUR KNOWLEDGE

SPACE FOR NOTES IS PROVIDED AFTER EACH CHAPTER FOR YOU TO ADD YOUR OWN "BITS AND PIECES" OF INFORMATION.

NOTES:

CHAPTER SEVEN
PACKAGING/ TRANSFER

KNOWLEDGE OBJECTIVES:
The rescuer should be able to...

- Describe the packaging procedure;
- Describe the use of a long spine board and rope sling in three different situations.

SKILL OBJECTIVES:
The rescuer should be able to...

- Package the victim for removal;
- Use the long spine board and rope sling to remove a victim lying on the front seat of the vehicle;
- Use the long spine board and rope sling to remove a victim from the floor behind the front seat;
- Use the long spine board and rope sling to remove a victim from underneath a vehicle.

CHAPTER SEVEN

PACKAGING/TRANSFER

In the event you have a suspected spinal injury, you may want to complete your survey before immobilizing the victim(s), as you may not be able to do so once the victim(s) is secured to an immobilization device.

Packaging begins when the freeing of the victim(s) is complete, and terminates when the injured person(s) are packaged and ready to be removed from the wreckage. It includes the following: the reinforcement of bandages and dressings that were placed on major wounds during initial emergency care efforts; the dressing and bandaging of lesser wounds that will be hidden by immobilization devices; at least the makeshift stabilization of fractures if the proper immobilization devices cannot be used, and the immobilization of the spine.

In critical patients, treatment of non-life or limb threatening injuries may need to be delayed until after transport begins.

Remember to remove any and all items that are bulky, sharp or in any way could harm the victim or interfere with securing the person to an immobilization device.

Removing an injured person involves much more than simply lifting and pulling the victim from accident wreckage. It must be accomplished in such a way that existing injuries are not aggravated and new ones produced. This is why the prior chapters dealt with creating working space and means of access and exit ways.

Injured persons can be removed from an upright accident vehicle in a number of ways.

An immobilized seated person can be removed through the adjacent door opening on a long spine board. A person who is lying on a seat can be removed on a long spine board or a scoop stretcher. A person who is on the floor of the vehicle can be pulled onto a long spine board with a rope sling.

Injured persons can be removed from a vehicle that is on its side with a long spine board and a rope sling. People who are piled on top of one another can be removed one at a time from the top down.

The use of the long board and rope sling works well in removing an injured person from underneath a vehicle that is on its wheels, such as the case of a car slipping off a jack and pinning the victim.

Regardless of the manner in which they were removed from an accident vehicle, the injured person(s) must be firmly secured to a rigid patient carrying device as soon as they are clear of the wreckage.

Long backboards, short backboards, K.E.D.'s, M.E.D.'s, Sherman vests, and scoop stretchers have all become tools of the trade. Yet, few units employ the long board and rope sling (Fig. 7.01 & Fig. 7.02).

For this reason, I would like to show their use in detail.

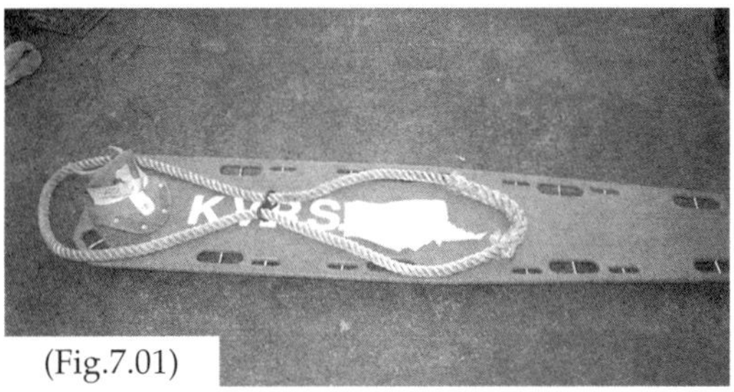

(Fig.7.01)

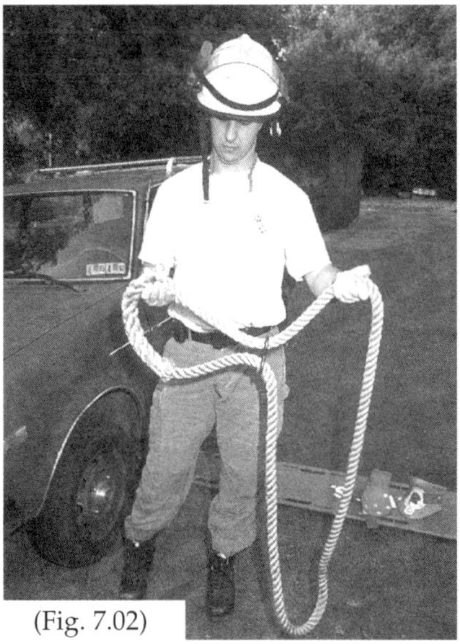

(Fig. 7.02)

Removing an Injured Person Lying on a Vehicle's Seat

Because of the victim's position, it's unlikely you would be able to secure him to an upper body immobilization device without a lot of movement. The victim can be pulled onto a long spine board, however, with a minimum of spinal movement.

*—Have your partner get into a position where he can apply a rigid cervical collar and support the victim's head.

*—Put the person in as anatomically straight a position as possible keeping the nose, neck and navel aligned (Fig. 7.03).

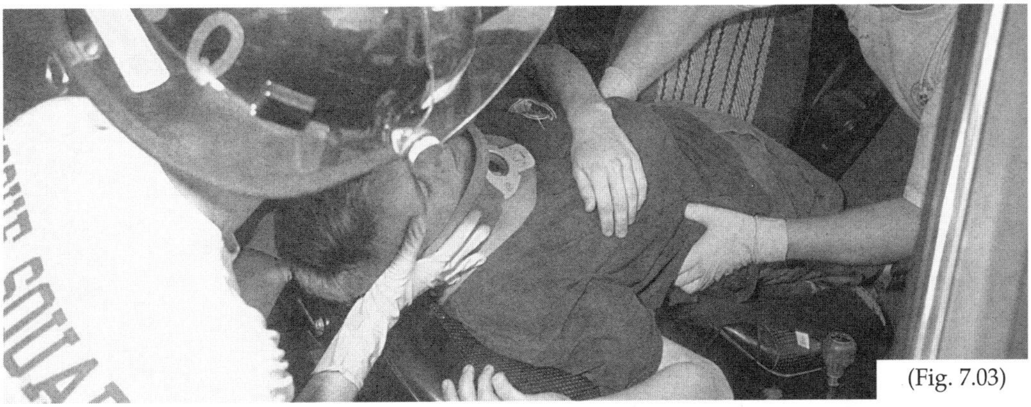

(Fig. 7.03)

*—While your partner supports the person's head and shoulders (in a slightly elevated position).

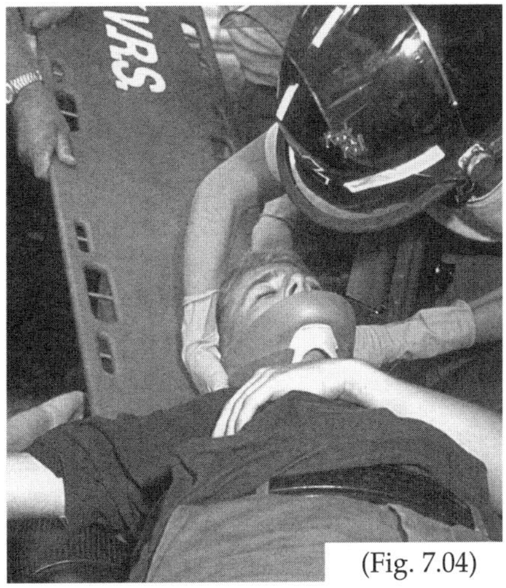

(Fig. 7.04)

*—Slide one end of the spine board between the person and the seat. You need to advance the board only to the point where the edge is beyond the shoulder blades (Fig. 7.04).

*—Lay the splice of the rope sling on the person's chest at the level of the armpits.

*—Work the sling under the person's arms so the rope is snug in the armpits (Fig. 7.05).

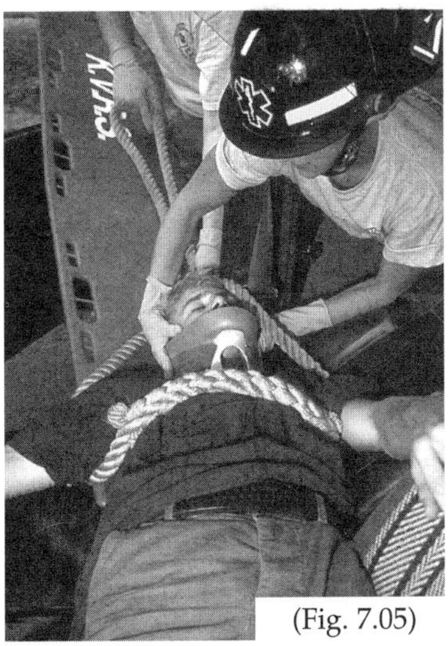

(Fig. 7.05)

*—Slide the adjustment ring behind the cervical collar so that the parallel parts of the sling will help support the person's head as he is being pulled onto the board (Fig. 7.06).

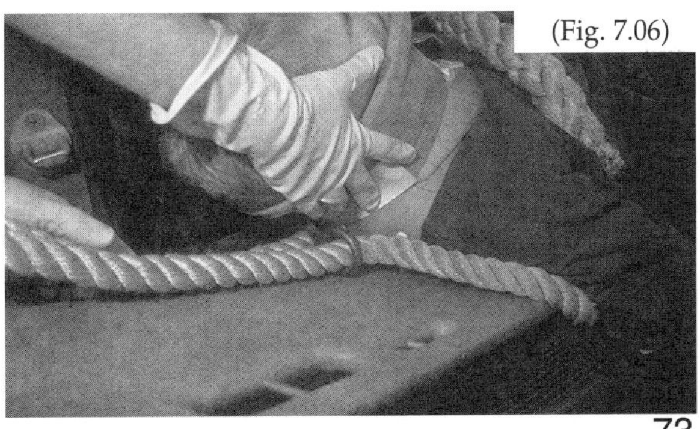

(Fig. 7.06)

*—Secure the person's hands together on his abdomen with a Velcro strap, a cravat, or a few turns of cling. This will prevent the arms from moving when pulling on the sling (Fig. 7.07).

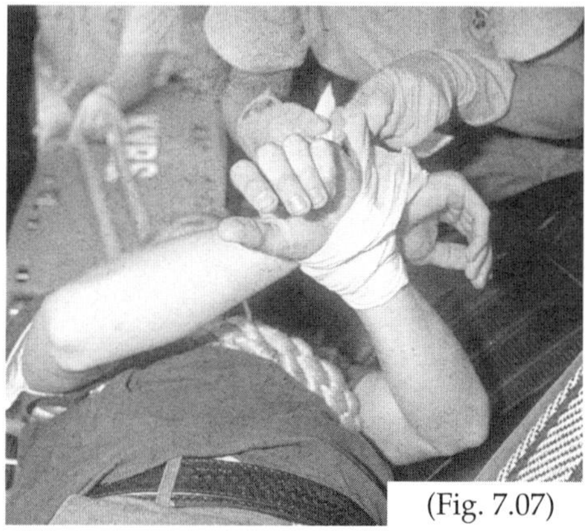

(Fig. 7.07)

*—While your partner holds the person in position, move to the end of the board.

*—Exert a smooth steady pull on the sling to move the person onto the spine board.

*—Keep your hands as close to the board as possible, to prevent lifting the person's shoulders from the board (Fig. 7.08, 7.09, 7.10).

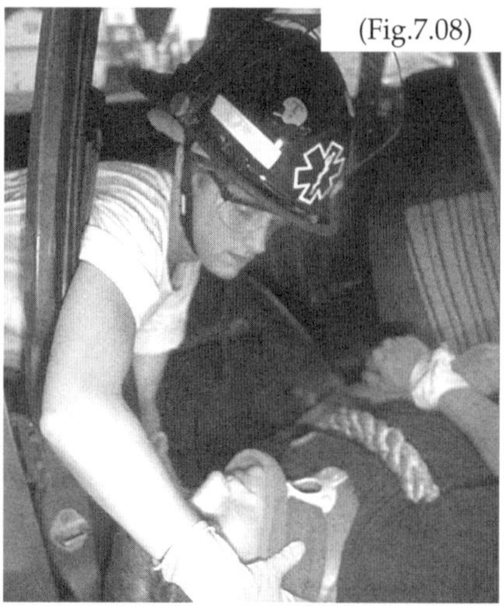

(Fig.7.08)

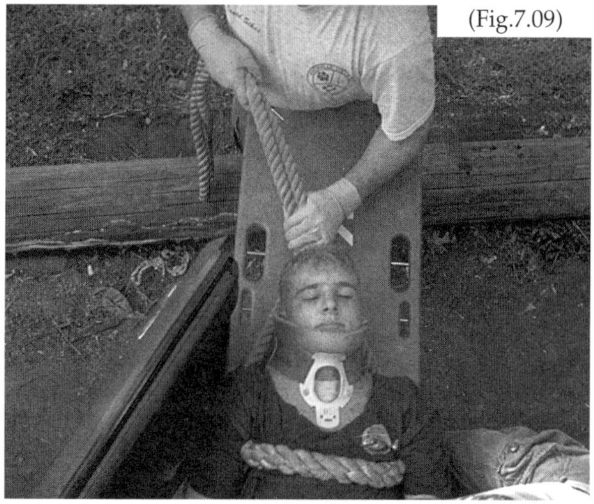

(Fig.7.09)

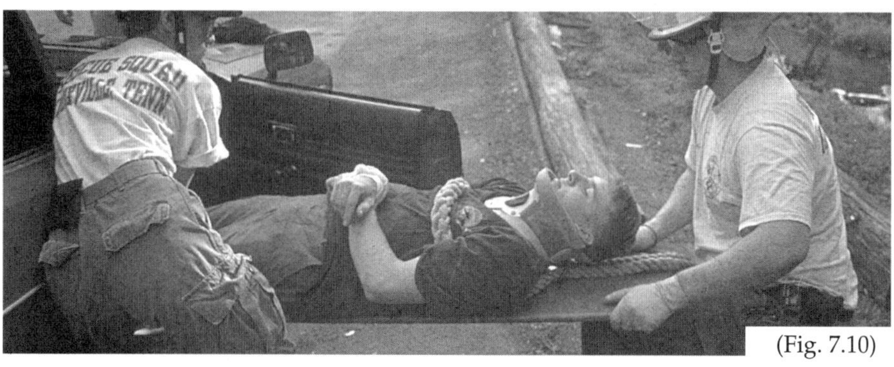

(Fig. 7.10)

*—Secure the person to the board and transfer.

Removing an Injured Person From the Floor Behind the Front Seat

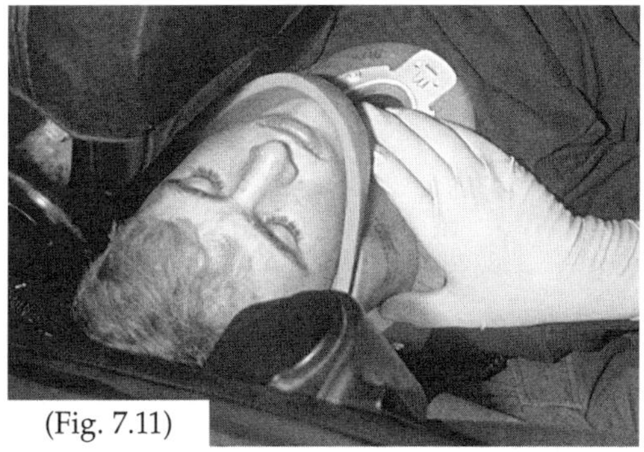

(Fig. 7.11)

*—Apply a rigid cervical collar (Fig. 7.11) and with the help of your partner, remove the rear seat. Most rear seats are easily removed by pushing down on each side while exerting rearward pressure.

Get the seat out of the vehicle. If the seat will not come out in the conventional method, do not waste time trying to out-smart it. Move on.

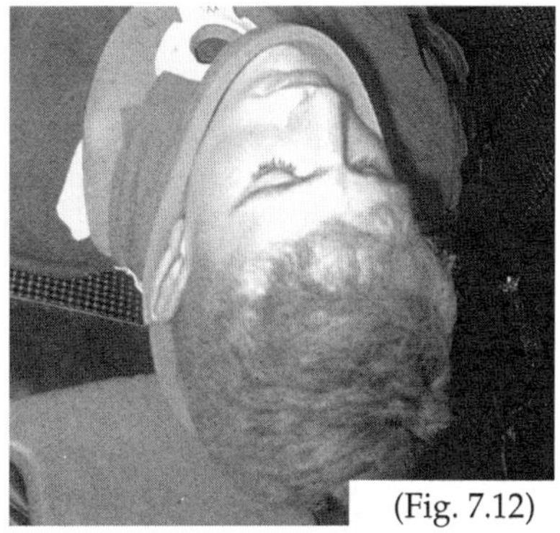

(Fig. 7.12)

*—While you straddle the person lifting the head and shoulders, have your partner slide the long spine board under the person far enough that it is beyond the person's shoulder blades (Fig. 7.12).

*—While your partner holds the board in position, lay the splice over the person's chest at the level of the armpits.

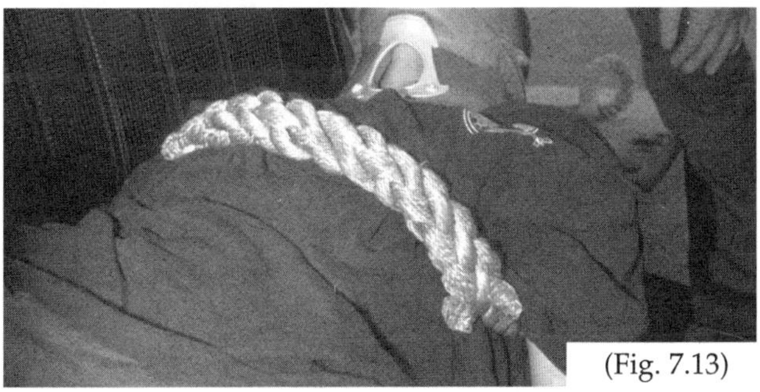

(Fig. 7.13)

*—Work the sling under the person's arms so that the rope is snug in the armpits (Fig. 7.13).

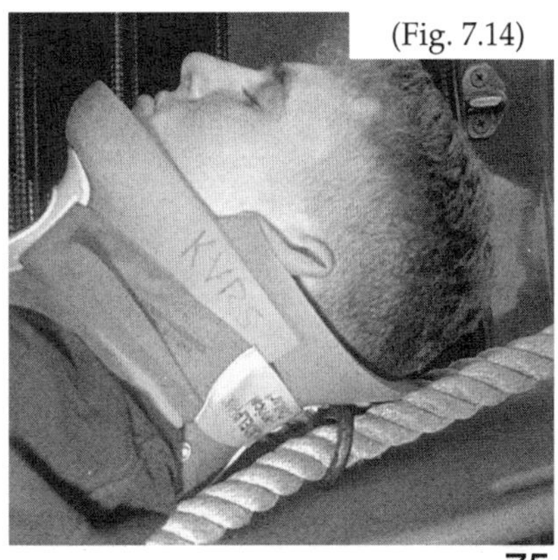

(Fig. 7.14)

*—Slide the adjustment ring along the rope toward the person's head and position it under the collar (Fig. 7.14).

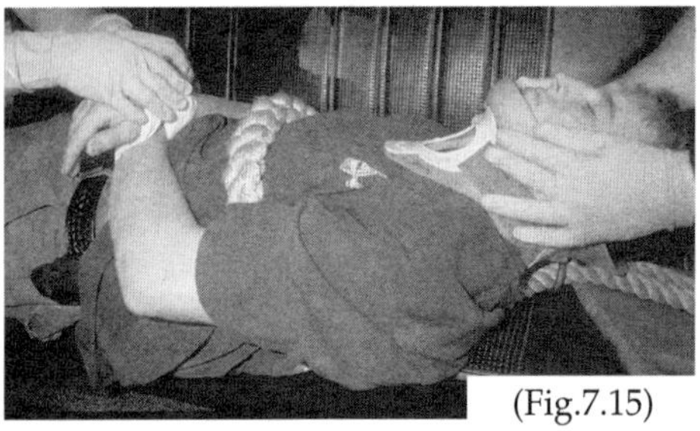

(Fig.7.15)

*—Secure the victim's hands (Fig.7.15).

*—While you support the victim, have your partner slowly pull the rope as you raise the victim's legs slightly.

*—Pull the victim onto the board keeping your hands as close to the board as possible. The adjustment ring will tighten up, thus supporting the victim's head (Fig. 7.16).

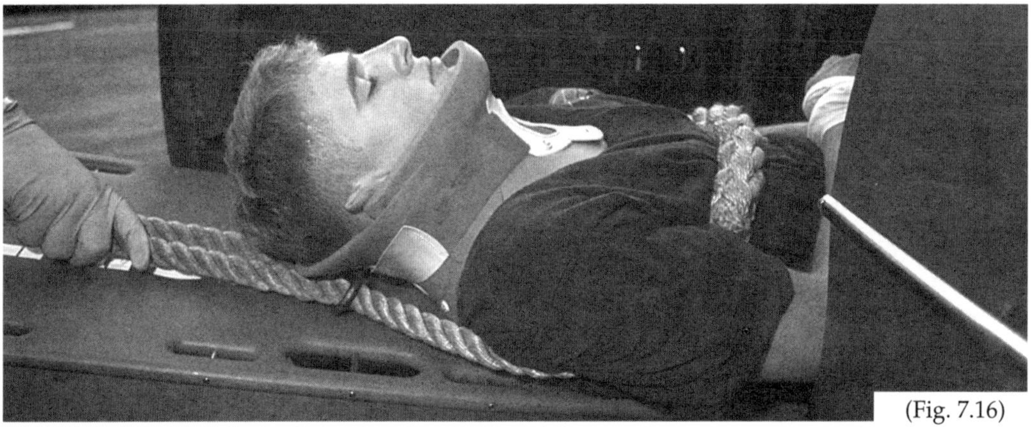

(Fig. 7.16)

*—Secure the victim to the board and transfer.

Removing an Injured Person From Underneath a Vehicle

The side of the car opposite the victims head is chocked and cribbed. The side you will work from is then lifted and cribbed. This method prevents the opposite side from pinning the victim as you lift on the head side. The victim should be placed in a rigid cervical collar (Fig. 7.17).

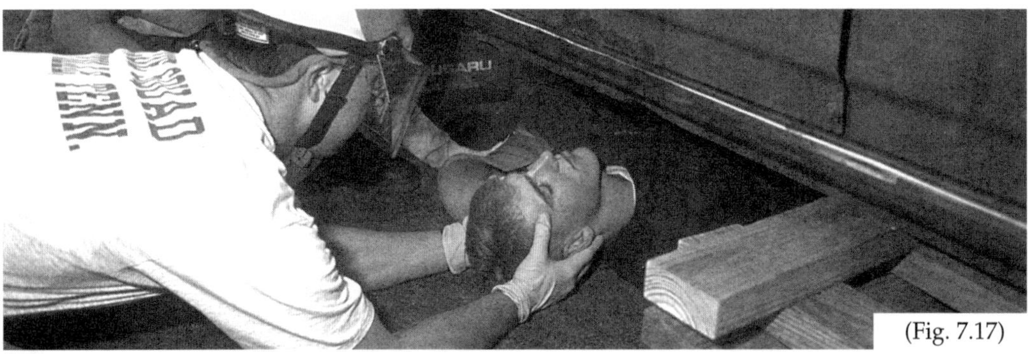

(Fig. 7.17)

Make sure there are no penetrating wounds or impaled objects in the chest or abdomen.

If the victim has a back injury or rib or extremity fractures, pulling him out by his arms, shoulders or clothing is likely to aggravate those injuries.

Using a rope sling to pull the victim onto a long board will involve minimal movement of body parts.

*—Lay the long spine board between you and your partner and close to the victim's head.

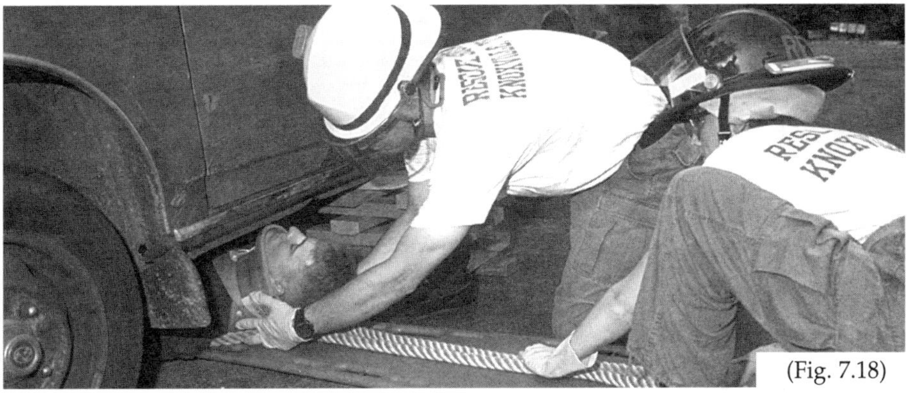

(Fig. 7.18)

*—While your partner raises the victim's head, neck and shoulders, slide the board under the victim's shoulder blades (Fig.7.18).

*—Gently lower the victim to the board and lay the splice of the rope sling on the victim's chest at the level of the armpits.

*—Work the sling under the arms so that the rope is snug in the armpits (Fig. 7.19).

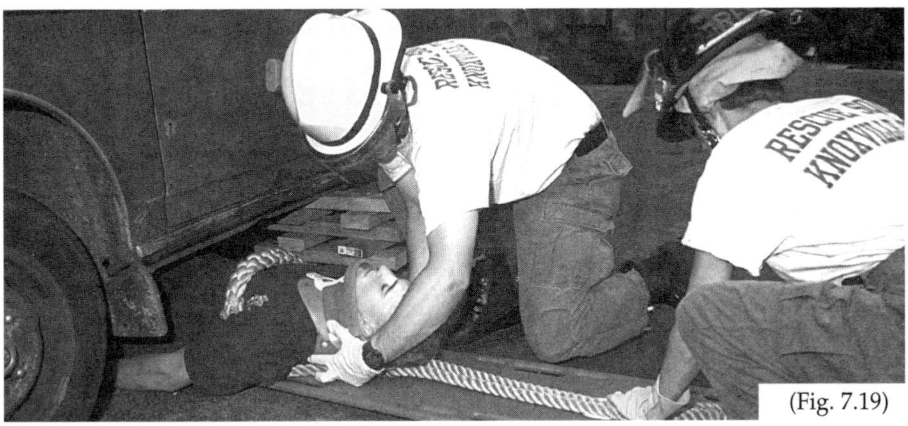

(Fig. 7.19)

*—Slide the adjustment ring along the sling until it is under the cervical collar supporting the victim's head (Fig. 7.20).

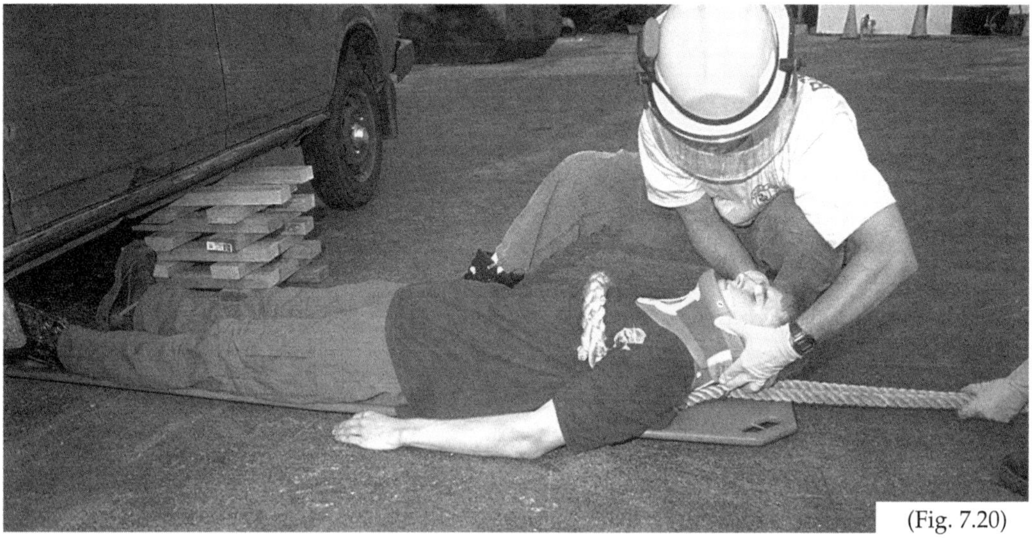

(Fig. 7.20)

*—Kneel at the end of the board and pull slowly. This position will allow you to keep the sling flat against the board (Fig. 7.20).

*—Secure the victim to the board and transfer.

KEY POINTS TO REMEMBER

*** The goal of spinal immobilization is to keep the spine in line.**

*** Align the "Nose - Neck - Navel."**

*** Move the victim along "the long axis", if not on a board.**

*** Always secure the victim to a spine board:**

With straps securing torso and legs.
With a neck immobilizer.

NOTES:

JOTTING DOWN IMPORTANT INFORMATION WILL HELP YOU REMEMBER AND EXPAND YOUR KNOWLEDGE

SPACE FOR NOTES IS PROVIDED AFTER EACH CHAPTER FOR YOU TO ADD YOUR OWN "BITS AND PIECES" OF INFORMATION.

HELP WANTED

Now that you have gone through the "ONE-WAY ONLY TECHNIQUES", I am sure you are beginning to pick up the idea that, "By gosh my partner and I can do more at the accident scene than stand around waiting for the BIG BOYS."

Not only can you do it, you may just be innovative enough to create new and even better ways to do the job.

There is nothing sacred written up to this point that will prevent you from being that person who will introduce a better, quicker, safer and perhaps revolutionary way to extend the "Golden Hour"!

To this end, I solicit your help.

If you have a procedure that can be used to the advantage of other Emergency Service Personnel, or if you know a bit of information that you feel should be included in this book, let us know. We will certainly consider including your contributions in future editions.

Send your comments to:

Rescue Training Consultants
Jim Gargan
444 Sandman Drive
Kure Beach, NC 28449

Thanks,
Jim Gargan

THE FOLLOWING RECOMMENDED LEARNING MATERIALS ARE AVAILABLE TO FURTHER YOUR KNOWLEDGE AND ABILITIES.

BTLS ACCESS INSTRUCTORS GUIDE

With 200+ Slides 1st Edition-1995
By
James B. Gargan
Roy L. Alson, Phd, MD, FACEP

An instructors guide with 200+ color slides is available exclusively through BTLS, International. The guide has been assembled to give point by point emphasis on the entire curriculum outlined by the BTLS ACCESS textbook.

Distributed by:

BTLS International

VEHICLE RESCUE

Second Edition, 1995
By
Harvey D. Grant
James B. Gargan

A Brady Book – Prentice-Hall, Inc.

A complete and in depth text that addresses techniques and equipment that may be used by all levels of rescue technicians. This text is designed to cover the needs of the basic rescue team, and advances to address the level of training necessary for the fully equipped rescue squad.

Distributed by:

Emergency Training Associates
&
Rescue Training Consultants